A Matter of Appearance

A Matter of Appearance

A Memoir

Emily Wells

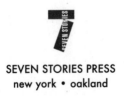

SEVEN STORIES PRESS
new york • oakland

Excerpts of this book appeared, in different form, in *The White Review*, in the *Los Angeles Review of Books*, and on Post45 Contemporaries. Thanks to those editors.

Selections from *White Ink: Interviews on Sex, Text and Politics*. Copyright © 2008 Hélène Cixous and Susan Sellers. Individual interviews, publishers, and contributors. Reprinted with permission of Columbia University Press.

Selections from *Winter Season: A Dancer's Journal* reprinted with permission from the University Press of Florida.

SEVEN STORIES PRESS www.sevenstories.com

Library of Congress Cataloging-in-Publication Data is on file.

ISBN 978-1-64421-314-8 (hardcover)
ISBN 978-1-64421-315-5 (electronic)

College professors and high school and middle school teachers may order free examination copies of Seven Stories Press titles. Visit https://www.sevenstories.com/pg/resources-academics or email academics@sevenstories.com.

Printed in the USA.

9 8 7 6 5 4 3 2 1

"Be very careful not to understand the patient.
There is no surer way of getting lost."

—JACQUES LACAN

PROLOGUE

Framed from a close distance, in aged monochrome: a woman, petrified in paroxysm, seated upright upon an iron hospital bed, etched against a black background. Her face is angled to catch the light, her back is arched, and hands are raised. She is dressed in a timeless white hospital gown, which has slipped off one shoulder and rests on her breast. She is otherwise unadorned. The photograph is labeled "Ecstasy," but the woman's euphoria is spiritual, not libidinous; something is absolving her of great pain, if only momentarily. She gazes

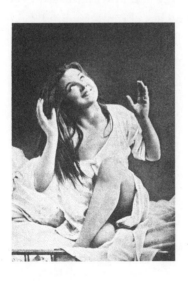

upward, beaming, like a woman who only has eyes for God. Either she is indifferent to being watched or she takes pleasure in it: she has to be captured. The phantoms of the image are not shown: just outside the frame is Doctor Charcot, with whom all healing starts. Perhaps her semiconscious gestures are borrowed, and if she is sensual, it is because she has been made so under his watchful eye. It may be that Charcot is instructing her in her bodily adjustments, rehearsing the physical manifestations of hysteria, the name he has given her symptoms, organic and provoked. Her virtuousness fissures slightly—a little thrill of self-importance, an oversight—as she, his favorite case, presents her body to him, to medicine. Charcot gives the signal—a snap of his fingers or a wave of his hand—and the woman loses hold of something. She sits up, confused. Everything is slipping away, everything that the photograph will later contain escapes her, and she is only a frightened girl, hair and arms in disarray, sitting in a hospital bed. It is as if she has abruptly realized she has been living an incorrect life. Charcot wants to cure the woman of her sickness, but it is already too late. The picture of a symptom, a medical riddle, is the form her life has taken.

Her name was Augustine Gleizes. She was the most performative, photogenic patient treated for hysteria at the Pitié-Salpêtrière hospital in late 1800s Paris, and thus the most famous. I discovered the images of her during one of my trips to the downtown Los Angeles library, where I like to write under the rotundas emblazoned with murals of scenes from California-history-as-stage-pageant. The artificial intention of going through the motions, blended with real intention and choices—even the absentminded choices of being about town—seemed decisive, so much so that a walk through the neighborhood could deliver purpose and, if I was lucky, the peace of mind that comes from true distraction.

When my joints didn't hurt too badly, I would select the appropriate combination of Schedule II pills from a small brass box; button my blouse as high as it would go; wrap myself in a large charmeuse silk scarf—the kind of *carré* you can't get at Hermès anymore, only at the estate sales of the old ladies dropping like flies around Wilshire—put on a wide-brimmed straw hat, heavy somehow, substantial, with an adjuster inside so it wouldn't blow away in the Santa Anas; and saunter the few blocks down Santa Monica Boulevard to the Metro station—driving while prone to fainting spells would have been a more dubious choice. The Metro would drop me off a short walk from the downtown library, an Art Deco building that, like most beautiful old buildings in Los Angeles, now seems pastiche, preserved in its celebration of public function.

Though I loved the walk, pain still seemed to come from everywhere—the air, the light—but I was foggily rooted on a cocktail of opiates and amphetamines. I didn't look sick; I looked like a young woman you'd expect to see in LA, one dressed in a way that suggested she didn't want to be looked at because of how often she was. People think that style is about enthusiasms, but like most matters of aesthetic consequence, it is actually a discipline of renunciations.

Wandering the stacks, I found Augustine Gleizes in a book of photographs of late-nineteenth-century hysteria patients who were treated by the neurologist Jean-Martin Charcot at the Salpêtrière hospital in Paris. She arrived there in 1875, just after turning fourteen. The discovery felt luminous, brightened by an idea. While the book offered little additional information about Augustine, I could tell immediately that the photographs of her were weighty in the manner of an allegory. Simultaneously, I felt the photographs taken during her tenure at the hospital might carry her imprint—the mark of her living, breathing body on the world.

After my library trips, walking back to the Metro under a tomato bisque sky, I would stop for an enormous coffee with real cream and perhaps sit for a bit with one of the other library frequenters, former academics too sick or too old or too home-less to continue working, writers who did not write. I would calculate my level of pain while I sipped, to see if I would be able to go out that evening. More than once, I had noticed that my pain was causing me to clench my teeth—a reaction I became aware of only when people at parties asked me for some of whatever drug they assumed I was on. But the day I found Augustine, I couldn't think of anything else and, instead, went straight home to spend more time poring over the book of her photographs. Perhaps women like myself, promiscuous pattern-seekers, go looking for ourselves in Augustine, that we might find in her a model for how we too can turn the landscape of mind and body into a black-and-white object from which we are detached, free to be posed and prodded without bother. Maybe we seek to connect our present with the past of another person, as if by venerating her, we grant dignity to our own suffering. It is tempting to reinterpret Augustine's illness and suffering as the political gestures of a feminist struggle or to ascribe her control over the photographic gaze—to look at her images and see power in her vulnerability—as a way to lessen the pain of bearing witness. While I hesitate to say Augustine's images invite projection, they are staggering, erupting with feminine excess. Somehow, Augustine's lack of composure defies the masculine logic of the images' documentary purpose. "But in truth I am only there as a photographer; I inscribe what I see," Charcot said of his confidence in the ability of the photographs to illustrate scientific problems. His photography director, Albert Londe, called the photographic plate "the true retina of the scientist." As if empiricism could ever be an entirely dispassionate act of looking and reporting. No, it is impossible to decipher Augustine's photos from that clinical distance.

As for the story of Augustine's illness, her life: like my own, it is about that which is unseen, that which cannot be extracted through images or medical measurements. Nevertheless, for some time, I have documented my symptoms, their ebbs and flows, their progressions, how ability trickles away. Always: nerve pain, inflamed joints, nausea, fatigue, oral ulcerations, general susceptibility to infection. Often: swollen lymph nodes, rashes, fever, dizziness, pins and needles, difficulty standing, muscle spasms, sensitivity to light, inability to digest food. Sometimes: hair loss, migraines, fainting. Symptoms are accompanied by correlating mental states (flashes of rage, confusion, despair, insomnia, dissociation) intermittently punctuated by brief euphoria when symptoms ease. To describe my body in terms of symptoms: it is as if it were not a body at all, but a broken-down, useless machine that cannot be restarted or repaired.

It is difficult to decide where to begin, because the story of the illness is not yet a story. To treat it as one seems to be the only way to gain the necessary vantage to know the secret I keep from myself, which is whether or not I can live with my pain. Perhaps, like Augustine, I will not be able to do so. But the sick person examining only her own suffering does so without a sense of history. My fundamental task is not to claim the tragic for myself, but to acknowledge those who make up the world of the sick; to create a space out of words for us to convalesce in together, to fight the ambient sameness of illness and the suspicion it brings with it: that what I write can only amount to the private dialectic of a frantic woman careening through life.

Augustine and her fellow hysterics have warned me of so much. *Passion* comes from the Latin root word *patior*, which, historically, refers to the time between the Last Supper and Good Friday, when Christ knew that one of the apostles would hand him over to be killed. Suffering is knowing what happens next.

I suspected that my body had its own inner life over which I had no physical control long before I encountered the photographs of Augustine. It goes back as far as I can remember, I should say, since one of my earliest childhood memories is watching a recording of a dance rehearsal filmed from the wing by another dancer's doting mother. Even now I can recall the sensation of sitting on the gritty sprung studio floor the week after the rehearsal, peering up at the outdated television in the corner, which seemed very high above me, as we were each asked to observe our performance and make notes on the areas we could improve. Then I remember the nauseating feeling as the excitement of seeing myself on-screen gave way to the realization that something had gone terribly wrong. Not with my performance—I danced well. The faster and more precise the movements, the more stoic and focused my expression grew. But as I made my exit from the stage, as soon as I was adequately shielded by the draped cloth of the wing, my face contorted into a grotesque wince. It was as though I had been waiting for this moment to surrender to an enormous, oppressive pain. I slid to the floor, crumpled, but did not hold onto or gesture toward any one part of my body: the pain seemed to come from everywhere, or nowhere. The woman holding the camera ushered the other girls away but allowed me to continue to tremble in the wing. I looked up at her pleadingly, both offering and protecting myself, and she finally seemed to understand that what she could do was grant me the small mercy of turning off her camera.

It may have been one of the earliest moments I preserved vividly, but as the next decade passed, I seldom returned to it. There was no need to: though this nameless pain continued interrupting my life, I was still able to insist upon a kind of belligerent sovereignty over my body, which had already been offered up to ballet, had already been spoken for. Sometimes, the pain became what I could describe as "unbearable," but so much of ballet feels unbearable; one is always finding new limits to what can be tolerated or sought. Dance isn't mind over matter; it's matter—flesh, bone, blood—over mind. Yet I still crumpled. Often. Anywhere.

Early in the course of an illness, symptoms might resemble affectations. My childhood was all blue fingers and toes, spells of being unable to eat because "flavors hurt," flu symptoms that persisted for months at a time. I always had a fever, *like a baby*, I was told. If these symptoms continue long enough without the discovery of the cause, people come to think of them as who you are. Immersed in the fantastical stories of ballet, I wondered when "the way I was" might become "the way I died."

In the ballet *Giselle*, a young peasant girl with a weak heart and delicate health is doomed to premature death by her love of dancing. Though her protective mother repeatedly warns her to remain still, Giselle can't help herself: she *has* to dance, and continues to flit around the stage. In a clichéd village scene, the other dancers stand around nodding, clapping, and gesturing toward her to indicate to one another that there is dancing happening at center stage. Ballet requires a great amount of pantomime—dancers gesticulate feelings and experiences instead of talking about them, a tendency I have found carries over into real life. Indeed, Giselle's fragility ends up being fatal: after she learns that her love interest is a nobleman and already engaged to another girl, she loses her mind—the mad scene is one of the most famous in all of ballet—yet maintains the impulse to dance, staggering around, grabbing at things that aren't there. In most modern renditions, the ballerina's hair is pinned in such a way that it will tumble down in tangled glory during this scene, so she can tug at it in a desperate, lionlike rage. Then Giselle's heart gives out, and she dies.

A young girl watching the ballet might believe that, in moments of terror and self-loss, she is supposed to do something with her hair. I was one of those girls. When I first saw *Giselle* being rehearsed by the older teens at my studio, I was overwhelmed by the sense that it was *my* story. Perhaps I already sensed that my love of ballet would harm me, or that I was dancing on borrowed time, but in all likelihood, I was too young and impressionable to have developed any immunity to the values embedded in the ballet: ritual, physical sacrifice, impossible beauty, and a story born of the mistreatment of women—or of a woman mistreating herself. Théophile Gautier, who cowrote the scenario for *Giselle*, was celebrated as an *abandonné* (one who yields or abandons oneself to a great artistic vision). It shows. The second act, which

I then thought was even more beautiful, follows Giselle into the afterlife, to the land of the Wilis, a group of ghostly girl-spirits who were betrayed by their lovers in life. The Wilis, clad in eidolic white tulle, are confined to haunt a graveyard and encounter mortal men only when they happen to wander through their domain by night.

They are a delicious, dynamic embodiment of collective female anger, indiscriminately seeking revenge on any man who comes their way before forcing him to dance until he dies of exhaustion. There are several different interpretations of the Wilis' backstory, though most agree that they are women who died before their wedding day or were left at the altar and could not find peace in their graves. From that point, readings differ: some choreographers and critics depict the Wilis as sexually frustrated (this might have been useful self-knowledge in my adolescence) or suggest that they find sexual fulfillment in their murders. The group's leader, the formidable Myrtha, either continues to condemn the women to their sexual frustration or provides them release and satisfaction with each dead man. Giselle begs the Wilis to spare Albrecht, the nobleman who misled her, but they insist that he is as guilty as any man and must die. Romanticism is often described as a rejection of popular morality in the pursuit of individual desire. When we interpret the Wilis in this way, it's noticeable that Giselle does the opposite, denying herself a sexually fulfilling experience in an attempt to save Albrecht. A dancer will deny herself anything for the story.

Now I wonder if dancers and the characters they portray abandon themselves to or for something. In the traditional stage production of *Giselle*, Myrtha ignores the girl's pleas for Albrecht's life. Male energy can run dry, but the wrath of women is infinite and unyielding. Albrecht deserves to die, Myrtha insists, and Giselle should relish his death with the rest of the scorned she-ghosts. But because it's a ballet, Giselle's merciful love rescues the nobleman, and she gets to rest peacefully in her grave. I've always wondered if a small but significant part of Giselle wanted to join the Wilis in their ravenous animus—the opposite of balletic virtue. The conditions of her choice feel modern: weaponize your ballet angelhood or lie, with your mercy and love of dance, in a coffin.

That's ridiculous, my own mother said of *Giselle*. *Why would you keep dancing if you knew it might kill you?* Still, I remained convinced that the most beautiful, meaningful pursuits would require correlating sacrifice. The older girls danced on shin splints and stress fractures. Some of them took secret "vitamins" that gave them boundless energy. If they gained weight, they dieted it away. The girls who couldn't see things that way, had bad feet, or gained the typical amount of weight during puberty—you can *see* more, Balanchine had said of his preference for thinness in his ballerinas—transitioned to modern dance, or became "civilians," the term some of us used to refer to nondancers.

One of my teachers had danced for Balanchine in his glory days at the New York City Ballet. She went by only her first name, perhaps in an attempt to mythologize herself in the same way she mythologized "Mr. B." When she spoke of him, her eyes took on a cultish, erotic glaze, which I mistakenly attributed to her love for ballet itself instead of her inability to get over having been touched by the Master. When she warned us that our aging would be an accelerated process—as though we were already, even as children, deteriorating in dog years—I felt let in on a secret that connected me with a grand tradition. But she was also a cautionary tale: as I imagined her preparing for her goddess-like descent on our class—brushing her wispy, waist-length white hair into a severe bun, wrapping her frame (which had no loose skin to indicate that she had ever gained weight or strayed from a balletic body) in tights and a chiffon skirt as though she were still a student—I felt unsafe from myself, as though I were quickly approaching a day when there would be nothing I could change about my life, either. Wanting might become an end unto itself.

In the old days, ballet dancers used bits of lamb's wool inside their pointe shoes, but by the time I was dancing, there were toe pads. From the outside, they look like socks, but there is a thin, valuable layer of gel cushioning built in. People often assume pointe shoes are made of wood from the sounds they make, but they're actually just layers of canvas and paper and glue, which make pointework quite painful, especially to young dancers, whose bones have not yet hardened. Our more traditional teachers, who wanted their girls to feel the floor through their shoes, to engage with the material matter of their art, abhorred these toe pads. As the civilians were weeded out, those of us who remained needed less padding in our shoes—just a little tape on the toes or some wadded-up paper towel did the trick. That taste, that desire to feel the floor, is what makes a dancer. The taste and the ability to know something many times over, forgetting and remembering and forgetting again.

In the 1860s, one of the last ballerinas of the Romantic era, Emma Livry, was famous for her portrayal of the title role in *Le Papillon*, a princess who is turned into a butterfly and burned when she flies into a lit torch. In 1862, Livry was rehearsing a mime part for an Auber opera when her skirt caught fire on one of the stage's gaslights. Costumes caught fire all the time—gaslights were everywhere—so ballet companies had begun fireproofing them. But Livry didn't like that the chemicals used stiffened and discolored the fabrics, and she refused the fireproof costumes. She spent months in the hospital as a result of her burns, but swore that if she were able to return to the stage, she would never wear the safer costumes, insisting that they were too ugly. She died in the hospital, and the remains of her charred costume can now be viewed in the Musée de l'Opéra, in Paris.

Group identity, suffering, sacrifice—it is no wonder that anywhere one looks, there are balletic relics and martyrs. Staunch exposés about the secret, ugly brutality lying beneath the calculated perfection of ballet are tedious because they're disingenuous. Ballet's cruel ferocity isn't a secret; it is at the heart of what ballet is—historically, in the popular imagination, and in the hearts of the tenacious, naïve children who pursue it.

Things could have been much worse, I often told myself. Tanaquil Le Clercq, the first American ballerina to be trained since childhood by Balanchine and the prototype for the thin, sleek Balanchine dancer, once told a friend that it had all seemed too easy: she had a scholarship to the New York City Ballet Company's feeder school, the School of American Ballet, at age eleven; was a principal dancer at NYCB at nineteen, and married Balanchine at twenty-three. Years later, while on tour in Europe, she caught polio and was paralyzed from the waist down. Of course, she at first wanted to die. Balanchine would pick her up from bed, place her feet atop his own, and dance around the apartment with her, propping her up—a hopeless endeavor. A year later, he choreographed *Agon*, a ballet containing a blunt pas de deux in which the male dancer controls and guides the legs and feet of the female dancer, poking and prodding and guiding, cruelly, erotically. When Tanaquil was fifteen, Balanchine had cast her in a onetime polio benefit at the Waldorf Astoria. He played an ominous character cloaked in black named Polio; Tanaquil portrayed his victim, falling to the floor at his touch, paralyzed. She was picked up and placed in a wheelchair, where she performed joyless arm movements until silver coins fell down upon her, "curing" her disease. When Tanaquil herself contracted polio, Balanchine believed that the performance had been an omen. It took him much longer than Tanaquil herself to accept that she would not dance again.

All I saw were stories—signs.

I played mental games with fate, listing tragedies that could ruin my life: the omens of harrowing ballet roles come true, a car accident, cancer, or a lifelong illness like Crohn's disease, from which my aunt suffered. Did I expect to feel a sense of control by imagining, in excruciating detail, each worst-case scenario? *That won't happen to you*, my parents insisted. *You're a Wells. A hard worker.* The casual association of debilitation with laziness provoked me to constantly reassure myself I was industrious: I could push through anything; enfeeblement would not happen to me—beneath pride there is always shame. My parents confidently distinguished between those who were poor and sick and failed by the cruel arrangement of society and those they thought to be a drain on the system, leeches who wouldn't do their part. To their disappointment, I failed to see any difference. Their judgments seemed to be made through a kaleidoscope of age, perceived choices, and appearance.

In a famous anecdote often told about Balanchine, now something of a cliché, a doting mother consults him about whether or not her daughter is suited for dancing. Mr. B. responds, "La danse, Madame, c'est une question morale." Dance as a moral consideration: while the abstraction is a bit maddening, it also seems predictive of who chooses to become a dancer. A young woman well suited to ballet considers sadism, masochism, and relinquishing her will to be moral questions. She is pleased to be an instrument.

In 1847, author Albert Smith published a "social zoology," *The Natural History of the Ballet-Girl*. While a widespread fascination with the seeming otherworldliness of ballerinas was common in the era, Smith instead painted a picture of dancers' lives full of bodily abuse, long hours in subpar conditions, and poverty, which gave them a sick appearance. But the physical demands were only the beginning. Smith wrote that the girls also looked ill because ballet roles emotionally manipulated them and overtaxed their feelings. The dancer must "express the most vivid interest in, and sympathy with, the fortunes, sorrows, or joys of the principal performers. Possibly, no other class of humanity is actuated by so many different sentiments in five minutes. Were the 'heart-strings' which poets write of, really bits of cord to pull the feelings into different positions, as the string makes the puppet kick its legs and arms, then you would see that those belonging to a whole Corps de Ballet are tugged at once." Because dancing in unison with the rest of the corps members does not allow for catharsis the way a principal role might, the ballet girl of the corps is left to feel too much.

Dance's easy historical association with madness did not help my case. In *Dance Pathologies*, Felicia McCarren argues that Smith's pathologizing of the ballet girl is indicative of how dance of the era addressed the discourses of literature and science, which became more pronounced as Romantic ballets moved toward wordlessness. Citing the purported connections among dancing, madness, and death in Romantic ballets like *Giselle*, she writes, "in a culture that views dancers as vaguely 'sick,' as Smith does—hysteria's myriad causes and symptoms seem a reasonable diagnosis." Both dance and medicine rely upon a normative concept of health, in contrast to which bodies are measured. While ballet responded not to medical theory or medical writing but, rather, to a general medical culture, it seems likely it informed the latter as well. Even Charcot, practicing what he called *médecine rétrospective*, noted the pathological association between hysteria and dancing in his discussion of medieval and Renaissance European dancing manias, claiming that hysteria and hystero-epilepsy played "a predominant role."

Romantic ballets like *Giselle* were used as political tools, inextricable from the pathologizing or sexualization of the young dancers. The noble Albrecht's betrayal of the poor peasant Giselle could be seen as a symbol of the harm done by the bourgeoisie, the very audience to which the ballet was presented. In his book *A Queer History of the Ballet*, Peter Stoneley writes that the tradition of *ballet blanc*, in which the female dancers are clad in white and tend to portray ghosts, nymphs, maidens, fairies, and other ethereal creatures, was likely seen as an erotic spectacle: when *Giselle* premiered at the Paris Opéra in 1841, the corps de ballet members who played the Wilis were expected to participate in a system of *prostitution légère*, endorsed by the Opéra, in which the women were connected with wealthy ballet patrons who made donations to the ballet in exchange for sexual favors or special attention from the dancers. The Palais Garnier even featured a *foyer de la danse*, an offstage arena designed to encourage encounters between high-paying patrons and the young dancers—a space that wives and male dancers were not allowed to enter. In the 1800s, these practices carried the fatal threat of syphilis, which McCarren believes was reflected onstage: the Wilis represented "many of the nightmares about female sexuality made evident in contemporary attitudes towards prostitution."

Nineteenth-century authority on hysteria Charles Leségue claimed that because its symptoms were too diverse and erratic, "the definition of hysteria has never been given and never will be." Indeed, for centuries, the history of the condition, as historian Mark S. Micale puts it, was "less linear than it is cyclical": one of the oldest surviving medical documents, from Egypt around 1900 BC, records bizarre behavioral symptoms in adult women believed to have been caused by movement of the uterus. This ancient Egyptian belief was adopted by classical Greek medical theorists of hysteria, who built connections between hysteria and an unsatisfactory sexual life. Ancient Roman physicians continued to associate hysteria with the female reproductive system, even if they did not believe the womb itself moved around the body. While Greco-Roman medicine viewed hysteria as an organic disease, Christian civilization in the Latin West created a punitive association of hysteria with demonic possession and witchcraft. By the Renaissance—the peak of the witchcraft craze in Europe—scientific and humanitarian efforts were made to renaturalize hysteria as a medical pathology. The seventeenth century marked a major shift: French royal physician Charles Le Pois argued that the pathology of hysteria was not tied to the womb but to the mind—a theory seemingly corroborated by seventeenth-century autopsies on hysterical patients that did not reveal any uterine abnormalities. Gynecological and demonological theories waned in the later seventeenth and eighteenth centuries in favor of a neurological model of the disease, though some physicians situated hysteria in the heart and pulmonary vessels or stomach. British clinician Thomas Sydenham formulated what could be called the first neuro-psychological model of the disease in 1681–82, asserting that the condition emerged from an imbalance in animal spirits between body and mind, typically from sudden intense emotional experiences like fury, fear, love, and despair. While Sydenham believed women to be more predisposed to hysteria due to a more delicate nervous system, he also described a similar condition in males. In the late eighteenth and early nineteenth centuries, the disease was re-eroticized: in a reversal of Hippocratic teachings, which associated hysteria with sexual deprivation, it was now blamed on sexual overindulgence. For the first half of the 1800s, French asylum doctors continued to disagree over the anatomical origin of the condition, and after the process of ovulation was discovered in the 1840s, a new "ovarian theory" remained prominent for the remainder of the century. Charcot, who was known as the "father of neurology," developed a broad model of hysteria as a disorder of the central nervous system during his time at the Salpêtrière from 1878 to 1893. Charcot sought, in some sense, to dignify the diagnosis of hysteria by providing a biological basis for the disease.

In 1885–86, Sigmund Freud studied at the hospital with Charcot after discussing the famous hysteria case of "Anna O."

(1880–82) with the internist who treated her, Josef Breuer. While Anna was in a hypnotized state, Breuer was able to trace her hysterical symptoms (cough, paralysis of extremities on the right side of her body, visual disturbances, neuralgia, hallucinations, and disordered eating, among others) back to past incidents that had caused emotional disturbances. After Breuer helped Anna bring to light the memory causing the psychic conflict, the correlating symptoms disappeared. In essence, Freud's development of the practice of psychoanalysis began as a theory of hysteria in contrast to Charcot's search for a biological explanation for the disease. Today, hysteria is primarily of interest to psychoanalytic, literary, and feminist theorists. No medical consensus has been reached on what hysteria is, why it is, where it is, or even if it is in the body. Yet, the condition continues to haunt contemporary diagnostic practice and the patients who must yield to it.

The idea that the body expresses itself in or through illness, or that illness can be caused by the mind, continues to haunt the language available to describe the experience of symptoms. When I fell ill, no one really called ballet girls "anorexic"— though it was obvious that many of us barely ate, for reasons both somatic and psychological, or simply to *be seen more*. It would have been like pathologizing the atmosphere. To most people around me, I was simply small, dramatic, and usually sick. In some sense, the knowledge was always there—that the thing that was wrong with me might have a name, that it might be wrong with other people, too. What was the point? I was skeptical of tidy diagnostic categorization even as I sought it. The issue is not that diagnostic categories are fake—or that "psychological" as opposed to "somatic" suffering is somehow less real—but that they are means to the end of accessing care, not ends in themselves. I didn't care what the name for my collection of symptoms might be, but I really, desperately wanted to stop fainting, to keep food down, to maintain a normal body temperature. I would come to think of the diagnostic process as a devil's bargain the sick must make with the market in order to receive the care necessary to survive.

I had internalized the idea that dance or medicine could say something about the body without words. Yet in silence, my body could be read as anything, optimal or pathological. How was I to come up with a way to interpret bodily semiology when physicians could not? In childhood, my illness was treated as a metaphor. I simply *felt too much*. I sounded crazy to civilians: a young woman who spoke about her body as though it were her essential stake in the world, an entity capable of moods entirely separate from her own. *Hysteric. Unable to control herself.* They were correct about that much.

Anecdotes I've forgotten about for years return as revelations: when I was no older than four, a cousin recounted to me how nauseated some rides at an amusement park made her feel. *Nauseated.* I hadn't heard the word before. I told my mother I learned a word to describe the stomach feeling I was always telling her I had. I can imagine her frustration that her child's states of distress were gaining articulatory power—my mother dislikes dramatic people—but, at the time, her exasperation confused me. Why wouldn't we want to know the word to describe what was wrong with us? I didn't yet understand that, just because something has a name doesn't mean people believe it's real—or that even conditions deemed to be real could be even less treatable than those dismissed as being "all in your head." And another thing: a family member noticed that I was always getting sick before "something important"— after travel, after sessions of particularly strenuous exercise. In hindsight: triggers of inflammation. As an adult, my adolescent overexertion would be granted the kind of explanatory capacity so often attributed to a poor diet or smoking cigarettes. Even a purely physicalist approach to interpreting disease grasps at individual blame; and they were *my* choices, after all. My parents were the farthest thing from stage parents. My mother encouraged my brother and me to be "well rounded" and chauffeured us to any activities our hearts desired; my father had hobbies; we took family vacations each summer. If I had oriented myself toward growing into a civilian more capable of harnessing the power of positive thinking, as they might have preferred, would my illness or the despondency I feel toward it look any different today?

That other Balanchine adage—about his wanting not the dancers who wanted to dance, but the dancers who *had* to dance—really meant something to us in those days. There was a world outside the tidy, homogenous life within the studio, but it was inconsequential. We all *had* to dance, but only I got sick and then couldn't. I thought, with calm abiding, *I feel so queasy; this means I am alive. I feel dizzy; this means I am a living being, that I can feel this, all these sensations.* I did not grow through puberty like civilian children. I commiserated with the other dancers on our constant fatigue, on the endless ministrations of the body, our worries so out of sync with those of other young people. We were living at an accelerated pace in which each year counted for more than an ordinary fraction of life.

This is probably when it started: when ballet became difficult. More than difficult: rather, extraordinarily painful. People described ballet as painful all the time, but I wondered if this was what it felt like for the other girls, if the simplest tendu sent searing pain through not only their pointed feet, but also their entire bodies. I wondered if they too had learned to angle their faces precisely during a grand jeté in such a way as to minimize any wincing. I assumed that this was what worthwhile endeavors felt like, that the ability to perform required suffering and sacrifice and ruin. I practiced what I called simply inhabiting, during which I would close my eyes, drive everything away, and drop into my body. I had muscle memory to fall back on, and this is what allowed me to get through class while I simply inhabited. Pain exists in the mind, and I knew I could be happy if I focused on a purely physical selfhood, one I spent several hours per day, six days per week, crafting. For a while, no one noticed how much harder things were getting for me, because I could appear to keep up, suffering the consequences later, alone. I got thinner; I was complimented. My hair thinned; I cut it. I got shin splints; I developed a taste for stimulants. My bony body remained pliable but became soft like an oil painting.

A dance teacher once described his own retirement and the bodily sensation of no longer being able to dance familiar movements as a loss of *muscular sanity*. Each of us looked down at an ailing limb as he said it.

When did it feel like a normal part of your life? I asked him.

He shook his head to indicate that it never did.

It was a term he might have read—though I doubt it—in an 1890 entry from Alice James's diary: "Owing to some physical weakness, excess of nervous susceptibility, the moral power passes, as it were for a moment, and refuses to maintain muscular sanity, worn out with the strain of its constabulary functions . . . it used to seem to me that the only difference between me and the insane was that I not only had all the horrors and suffering of insanity but the duties of doctor, nurse, and straight-jacket imposed upon me, too." In this same entry,

Alice references a paper by her brother William, titled "The Hidden Self," in which he writes that the hysteric "abandons part of her consciousness because she is too weak nervously to hold it all together." William believed the theories emerging out of the Salpêtrière that the abandoned part of the hysteric's consciousness "may solidify into a secondary or subconscious self" and that hypnosis could be used to "make her give up the eye, the skin, the arm, or whatever the affected part may be." Alice seems to have believed in this conception of hysteria, too, but often, the way she describes the cognitive aspects of her condition feel more akin to the sluggish "brain fog" that so often accompanies chronic illness: "When the fancy took me of a morning at school to *study* my lessons by way of variety instead of shirking or wiggling thro' the most impossible sensations of upheaval, violent revolt in my head overtook me so that I had to 'abandon' my brain, as it were . . . conscious and continuous cerebration is an impossible exercise and from just behind the eyes my head feels like a dense jungle into which no ray of light has ever penetrated." Alice's mother believed her to be suffering from "a genuine case of hysteria." As my symptoms continued to be interpreted as a lack of "nervous togetherness," I began to wonder if I might be, too.

My mother attacked the diagnostic process with all the deliberation of a nosediving dolphin. Blood was tested. Everything was scanned. I had no STDs, no mono, no epilepsy, no detectable viruses. A rheumatologist found no reason for my joints to be as they were. A primary physician looked at my blood and found slight anemia and vitamin B and D deficiencies, but nothing that should have been causing my long list of symptoms. A neurologist scanned my brain and found no reason for me to be dizzy so frequently. A gastroenterologist instructed me to keep a food diary in order to troubleshoot what might be causing the ulcers along my digestive tract. I updated that diary with religious devotion. I narrowed my daily food intake to cucumber, ciabatta, herbed mayonnaise, and a sleepy sheet of lettuce.

Easy, the gastroenterologist said after examining the food journal. *Nervous stomach.*

This does not explain any of the other symptoms, I reminded him.

As a doctor, he knew this. He offered me more painkillers. While I was fortunate enough to have access to medical troubleshooting, my body was categorically deceitful.

A common image of me from those years: I'm sitting on an examination table, wrapped in a paper gown in those insipid colors chosen specifically for women—lavender, maybe. I'm already suspecting that the brutal heat through each muscle, each joint, and in my blood itself will not be made legible through any conducted diagnostics. At each appointment, a nurse writes down my details in order of increasing incrimination: a young woman, a former ballet dancer (*control issues, short career*), experiencing recurrent episodes of fainting (*restricted eating*), nausea for extended periods of time (*histrionic*), sourceless pain everywhere (*performative*), rashes (*neurotic*), sleep paralysis (*a benign condition*). The nurse would ask me to rate my pain on a scale of one to ten. Each time, I'd hesitate, unsure of how to turn a sensation into a number. Should I have said nine and risk confirmation of my suspected inclination toward hyperbole, or four, and risk being misunderstood? Sometimes, the nurse then asked if I was anxious, which I was—anxious about what everyone else seemed to see: that it was a matter of anxiousness, not my body. I was anxious about being anxious without language to express what the body felt, the necessary crossroads of breath and text that might lead this suffering to the small mercy of a name. Or, in a confluence of visual data and psychology, she'd ask if I thought I was fat, or make an asinine comment about my thinness. I would explain, with the saccharine cadence one might use to speak to a child, that I ate all I could but that "the flavors hurt." Dry arugula met me with a shock of spice; I was pricked by the harshness of cilantro in a bowl of bland rice noodles. Hunger pangs, I would explain, were often easier to bear than the searing pain that followed soon after a flavor, or than the inevitable vomiting, diarrhea, and nosebleeds. She would write something down, furrow her brow, and ask how my periods were (*rare*). Had I tried protein shakes?

I'd sit there in the stupid gown, huddled and cupping my blue fingers around the warmth of my breath, and wait for the doctor. Dancers, I thought, were ideal patients: compliant, receptive to critique, and pleased to solve problems through bodily manipulation. I would look down at my body as if for the first time and try to see if there was anything that might indicate a problem to an outside eye. Aside from some tragedy behind my thinness that could be guessed at, or the bruises that perpetually sprinkled my arms and legs, no matter how careful I was moving through the world, or the general malaise of being a young woman, already working so hard, already *so tired*, I didn't look sick.

The doctor would come in and scan my chart while I disappeared. If he asked what I thought was going on, I would think it was a positive beginning: to be granted this authorship over my body. I always brought notes about recent symptoms on index cards, the same ones I used to memorize the minimal amount of information necessary to do well in school. They featured new sources of pain (*light, cold, heat*) scrawled in pencil, newly infected body parts (*fingers hurt the most*) or new observations about a correlation between diet and ulcers. As I spoke, I would often be struck by the pity in my own voice, as if I were speaking about some other unfortunate person in a state of undeserved catastrophe. It is hard, perhaps impossible, to contemplate one's medical legibility—the chasm between suffering and what can be found to be wrong—without self-pity. Pity slips through when we are told we will remain impenetrable to ourselves. I'd try to explain whatever my most recent incident or symptom was, speaking slowly and calmly: *This time, my most recent fainting spell was not provoked by anything in particular. It happened after a pleasant lunch with friends on the patio. When I rose to clear my plate, I felt the flurry of clichéd symptoms that occur before losing consciousness: the room spun. I felt a weightiness throughout my body and the sensation of being pulled downward before blacking out, hitting my head, and receiving a minor concussion. Since then, the sensation of being pulled downward has not left me. I've lost my sense of balance and endured an unrelenting migraine and ringing in my ears.*

Sometimes, while recounting my symptoms, I would get uncharacteristically flustered; would mumble, cough, skip some of the items listed in my notes. (*It feels like there are knives flowing through my blood, and all my blood is rushing to my head.*) Then, the doctor would clear his throat, explain that my cranial MRIs, assisted by vibrant dye dripped into my bloodstream in the days following my fainting episodes, had come back normal, that there was no reason to assume anything was wrong with my brain or anything else and that they were running out of tests that could be run. Always, it concerned him that I seemed anxious, which he could offer me something for. Always, he reminded me that women, especially women under a great deal of physical or emotional stress, often do not realize they are experiencing anxiety or that this anxiety is what causes ailments that seem physical in origin. Always, he said that our minds and bodies interact in mysterious ways. There was never anything conclusive. Once, I asked what I really wanted to know: *If all my symptoms persist while the tests continually, conclusively show that nothing is wrong with me, does this not suggest that it is the diagnostic process that is inadequate?*

Maybe, he said, *but in the absence of an observable cause, the overwhelming likelihood is that what we're dealing with—we!— falls within the realm of psychiatry.* If whatever was causing my symptoms had an organic cause, it would show up on tests. This was the rule by which he had to practice medicine, he told me. *Maybe it's the rule that is broken, then*, I said under my breath. He prescribed an antidepressant.

Sometimes I pleaded, knowing fully that objecting to the diagnosis that it was all in my head would only reinforce his belief that it was all in my head.

Surely, this pain, this physical *pain, cannot come from anxiety alone*, I said.

If the doctor was generous, he'd ask how often I was in pain.

Even today, while I am in considerably more pain considerably more often, I wonder if I know the answer to this question. One day, I might find myself feeling adequate and relatively positive; the next, I will not be able to leave bed, giving in to a pain I can't verbalize. From a medical perspective, my self-conception is unreliable at best. I would tell myself it was fine for the doctor to cushion the air with banal assumptions. I understood that his interest was restricted to the zones stipulated by the form he was filling out and that for me to offer information that could not be put into that form only made both of us uncomfortable.

To ask, to *beg* the doctor to explore my situation, to ask him to inhabit my bewilderment, was pointless. If your scans do not contain the necessary indicators that lead to diagnosis, they will be thought to reveal similarities between you and those who allegedly only *imagine* themselves ill. If you present as composed, poised, you will seem too *well* to be suffering as much as you say. If you present as distressed, the distress serves as an easy scapegoat, the reason you feel so unwell. A plea bargain is as good as it gets.

Philosopher and art historian Georges Didi-Huberman writes, "All the efforts of pathological anatomy in the nineteenth century were not only directed toward configuring the illness through a distribution of symptoms, but also and above all to subsuming this configuration: to *localizing the essence of the ill*. The sign of the illness became less the symptom than the lesion." Symptoms prevail.

"One has a greater sense of intellectual degradation after an interview with a doctor than from any human experience," Alice James wrote in her diary.

Charcot's disciple Désiré Bourneville noted that "the hysteric always seems to be outside the rule." She might suffer from seemingly incongruous symptoms, like stupor and hypersensitivity, anorexia and bulimia, constipation and diarrhea, depression and profound intelligence (once again, it is the rule that strikes me as inadequate). Thus, hysteria became known for its ability to mimic countless other illnesses. Charcot had become famous as a neurologist for his ability to find the "essence" of a disease visually—first, by identifying common patterns of patients' symptoms and, then, by overseeing postmortem dissections of their brains, seeking a common structural abnormality. This "clinico-anatomic" method sought to ensure he would not be led astray by the specificities of individual cases. Charcot's job, as he saw it himself, was to turn disarray into classification. He identified two kinds of hysterical symptoms: permanent physical defects that, as a dig, he called "stigmata"; and periodic fits that could come on spontaneously or when a patient was surprised, distraught, or scared. Charcot believed that with better microscopes and scientific techniques, he would eventually be able to find the abnormality of the brain that was surely the source of the hysteric's symptoms. But after centuries of inquiry, we still do not know what caused them. There was certainly a culture shared among the "career" hysterics—our illnesses are always social. One of them, Marie "Blanche" Wittman, too unpredictably violent and disorderly to be of clinical value (though her angry outbursts may have been a result of her addiction to ether, a common anesthetic used at the hospital), was transferred from the hysteria ward to a cell in the insanity ward for over seven months as punishment. When, seven and a half months later, she returned to the hysteria ward, where patients were offered more freedom and privileges, she worked to become a model (hypnotizable) hysteric and was featured prominently in Charcot's demonstrations. It's easy to see why a young woman resigned to spending her life at a hospital might try to climb its ranks through imitation, but a predictable assemblage of symptoms and their progression had already been established as requirements for something to be classified as a disease by medical pioneer Thomas Sydenham in the seventeenth century. Even subtracting symptoms that might be explained as imitative or social, like the attacks—many hysterics were indeed housed with epileptics when they arrived at the hospital, and Charcot's famous demonstrations there tend to be read today as theatrical performances—what of the others? Charcot himself claimed that the hysterics' fits and hallucinations were too intense not to be authentic. It all raises the question: if Charcot was looking for a brain lesion, proof that the hysterics' condition was rooted in biology, not the mind, why was the diagnostic process so obsessively visual, with hysteria symptoms staged under hypnosis in darkrooms and amphitheaters opened to observation? As cultural historian Cristina Mazzoni puts it, "[Charcot's] clinic ends up resembling its object of study, be it an artistic text or hysterical woman." (Was I perhaps drawn to the hysterics' images because they offered some false hope that pain could be *made* visual?)

The pathologizing of Giselle's sexual "deviance" and her "madness" provided the basis for Swedish choreographer Mats Ek's poststructuralist reworking of the ballet, which premiered in 1982. In this rendition, Giselle propositions Albrecht, indicating to him that although she is not fertile, she still has sexual desire. Albrecht's requited desire stems from his exchanges with Giselle rather than from a myth surrounding her figure. Instead of dying of a broken heart, Giselle is banished to a mental asylum. Thus, the death of her body at the end of the first act can be read as synonymous with the loss of her sanity. The second act takes place in an asylum, where the Wilis are recontextualized as Giselle's fellow patients: they will never be mothers, will only ever be frustrated. With nothing to control their desire, they are ruled by sexual impulsivity. Myrtha is a nurse reminiscent of Nurse Ratched in *One Flew over the Cuckoo's Nest*. The surreal sets feature dismembered pieces of the female body scattered across the asylum walls. In a maneuver akin to that of the fainting husband in Charlotte Perkins Gilman's *The Yellow Wallpaper*, Albrecht follows Giselle in succumbing to madness.

Ek's isn't an emancipatory vision, but it does seem to hold culture and, by extension, ballet culture more accountable for what it does to women. When asked if he considered his staging of *Giselle* to be deromanticized, Ek responded, "That depends on what you mean by 'romantic.' If you mean 'pretty and sweet,' well, no, they're not part of it. But if you mean what 'romantic' signified from the beginning—something wild and illogical, something to which you can't respond with your reason—then, absolutely, this is a romantic ballet." His answer is akin to the surrealists' post hoc obsession with the hysterics; or to Lacanian psychoanalysis's defense of hysteria as a condition capable of entertaining dichotomies. When the body itself is wild and illogical, it demands to be met on these terms.

If we are to accuse hysterics of imitation or susceptibility to suggestion, we ought to be sure of what it is they might have been imitating. Dance scholars often highlight the similarities between the movements of hysteria, epilepsy, and catalepsy and the seemingly automatic, involuntary movement's symbolic representation of the body's triumph over reason, bringing with it a fundamental lack of control. Whether the dancer or hysteric identifies with her movements or mimics those of others is not clear; nor is the difference between the two.

The era in which Charcot worked marked a turn after which behaviors formerly thought of as religious expression were recast as symptoms of illness, though Charcot's obtrusively visual diagnostic process certainly reinforced the casual association of hysteria with mysticism. He confidently proclaimed as hysterics women previously thought to be possessed by demons (or, occasionally, canonized as saints). Just before his death, he published a paper on "Faith-Healing" in which he diagnosed Francis of Assisi and Teresa of Ávila as "undeniable hysterics," and in *Les Démoniaques dans l'art* (1886), a collaboration with graphic artist Paul Richer, he reinterprets a series of illustrations depicting demonic possession and religious ecstasy as portraying symptoms of hysteria. Freud's colleague Josef Breuer, who dubbed Teresa of Ávila the "patron saint of hysterics," observed that hysteria patients' poses often seemed to be modeled on depictions of Teresa. Self-starvation and mutilation of the flesh, even when carried out by a religious patient professing penance, were relegated to the list of hysterical symptoms. In a sense, the medical world sought to "save" the women in a capacity formerly left to the Church, a practice largely perpetuated by the assertion that hysteria was a purely biological disease. In a short story by Guy de Maupassant (who had viewed Charcot's Tuesday lectures at the hospital), a character airs their grievance: "[Charcot] has set forth some nervous phenomena which are unexplained and inexplicable; he makes his way into that unknown region which men explore every day, and not being able to comprehend what he sees, he remembers perhaps too well the explanations of certain mysteries given by priests." By 1883, the beds in the Salpêtrière, previously named after saints, had been renamed after scientists. But the women treated there were still sick.

Many suggest that the hysterics chose life at the Salpêtrière for reasons similar to their predecessors who chose convent life: because it was a more tolerable existence, a respectable alternative to marriage. When Teresa of Ávila entered a Carmelite convent just outside the city's walls in 1535, her decision to do so was somewhat informed by her desire not to marry and be stuck at home as her mother had been. The Convent of the Incarnation was likely a better place to endure the countless symptoms she might have experienced in the outside world: the rules were fairly relaxed and the sisters wore elegant habits; lived in large, comfortable rooms; and received guests regularly.

In the convent or the hospital, hysterics and mystics found a place where their symptoms were received and given a framework in which to be interpreted. When Teresa was nearly forty and finding it difficult to pray, she experienced what she believed to be a mystical union with God before an image of a wounded Christ, "that He was within me, or that I was totally engulfed by Him." She devoted herself to a theology of mysticism and asceticism informed by similar episodes, which occurred constantly thereafter. Most curiously, it is in this state of rapture that she experienced healing from her symptoms—or, at least, the symptoms she considered to be the result of illness. She wrote prolifically during this period of her life, and her resulting autobiography has also come to be read as an exceptionally rare and detailed medical record of the time.

In *Preliminary Materials for a Theory of the Young-Girl*, Tiqqun wrote, "A pandemic similar to the one we see today among Young-Girls emerged at the heart of the Middle Ages among the saints. Against the world that would reduce her to her body, the Young-Girl opposes her sovereignty over her body. In the same way, the saint opposed the patriarchal mediation of the clergy to her own direct communion with God; she opposed the dependency through which THEY would have liked to keep her to her radical independence from the world."

Long after their bodies are lost to history, we never stop obsessively trying to diagnose these women in *our* time's language. When the diagnosis of hysteria was no longer considered viable, secular historians reinterpreted Teresa's symptoms as likely to have been caused by temporal lobe epilepsy. Others levy a diagnosis against all these women like a condemnation: dramatic imitation or mass psychogenic illness. Elaine Showalter writes that hysteria imitates "culturally permissible expressions of distress" and that, over time, these articulations have changed with the cultures surrounding them into epidemics believed to be psychogenic, like chronic fatigue syndrome, Gulf War syndrome, multiple personality disorder, and satanic ritual abuse. But, reading Teresa's autobiography as a teen, I did not know this, nor had I formed a healthy skepticism about the historical evolution of diagnostics, what diagnostics are for. I did not think about the likelihood that Teresa had suffered from an unknowable combination of organic illness, religious ecstasy, and revolt against circumstance. I simply believed that she experienced her illness as she said she did: God roused her soul, and the suppression of basic physical urges corresponded with the relief of symptoms, so she could be unified in rapture with God. It felt important to believe what a woman had said about her own life.

Another patient of Charcot's, the French novelist Alphonse Daudet, wrote, at the beginning of notes on his disintegration from syphilis, a common Greek tag that translates to "Suffering is instructive." Daudet observed his fellow sufferers at Lamalou, a thermal station in southern France preferred by those recovering from (or sinking farther into) syphilitic illness. (The discovery that neurosyphilis had a physical basis had fueled Charcot's belief that other forms of mental illness and "abnormal" behavior would eventually be explained by brain pathology.) Many Lamalou syphilitics were farther along in their illness than Daudet, who used his observations of their symptoms to predict how he might fare himself. His friend Edmond de Goncourt wrote in July 1880, "Poor Daudet, who is haunted by an idée fixe: the fear of degradation, and the physical shame which paralysis entails. And when you try to reassure him, he tells you that he has studied the progression of his disease among his fellow-sufferers at Lamalou: he knows what will happen to him next year, and what will happen to him the year after." Most chronically ill people don't have such specimen comrades to help predict how they might fare.

The thinking body is all that remains of my time in ballet. My memory is littered with holes—or, rather, certain details are out of order in my mind: when my bones started to splinter, when I gave in to certain choiceless clichés, when I knew I would be spat out in fury but danced on anyway. I couldn't understand back then why some teenagers left ballet. *It's to save our bodies*, one of them told me. I scoffed.

Contempt was my first mistake.

My second mistake was pride. When a ballet teacher pulled my mother and me aside one afternoon and gently suggested I consider taking a meeting with an acting agent, I understood that my simply "inhabiting" wasn't cutting it—I was destined to be a civilian. I didn't take a breath the entire time she spoke. My notoriously harsh ballet mistress was trying to tell me, in the most generous way, that my time with her was waning. Ballet careers are rare and punishing, and it was already resolutely clear that I would not have one. The summers I'd spent in acting classes held at ballet intensives—*Loosen up and have some fun!*—and the overlap of skills used in ballet meant that acting might have been an easy transition, and it certainly would have earned better money and been less strenuous on my body. None of this mattered. Losing ballet meant losing the illusion I held closest: that all my physical suffering was *for* something—ballet, beauty, a Mr. B., a god, or a Charcot. If my body's usefulness as a vessel was about to run dry, I believed that the only relief I might find would come from transcendence from my boiling flesh-prison. I began to see my body as not a temple but an escape room.

I have never found a version of life that expresses itself like dancing, but sometimes, in a dream, I am able to recall what the pleasure of it felt like in my body, and I am briefly consoled.

I swore to forget the sick girl and speak of her to no one. I wanted to stop thinking about her entirely—her confusion; her harshness toward herself and her surroundings; the conflict between the world and how she wanted it to be, the manufactured perfection of a well-executed performance; her conflation of matters of taste with laws of nature; her inability to provide a satisfactory account of the chaos enveloping her. But I have never managed to forget. Years later, all my fiction was written toward her, toward her posturing, her tendency to act like she knew what she wanted before she did. Obeying the instinct to immerse myself in that part of my life once more, to investigate a medical event devoid of evidence, was a daunting prospect. The narrative has lugged me along in directions I have not chosen: toward Augustine Gleizes, toward martyrs, and now toward my unproven body and the secrets it harbors.

"Hysterics suffer for the most part from reminiscences," Freud and Breuer wrote in *Studies in Hysteria*.

The antidepressant medication prescribed by the neurologist who could find no organic cause for my fainting spells did not resolve my dizziness or fainting. It made me more nauseated, doubled my pulse rate, worsened my insomnia and subsequent night terrors, and made me feel as though an electrical current were traveling around my body just under my skin. When I called the neurologist's office to let him know that I would stop taking the medication—dangerous to do abruptly, but no one informed me of this—I was treated as though my resistance to continuing were just another symptom of mental unwellness.

You wouldn't hesitate to take medication if something were wrong with your liver or your heart, he said to me, as if any of my symptoms had been conclusively traced to my mind, as if I had not entered his office beseeching him to find what was wrong with any organ so that it might be treated.

I asked him, *What if, hypothetically, I continue to take the medication, but do not feel physically any better?*

He said that we would then try a different antidepressant, or a booster medication. We would keep trying medications to treat my mind until one of them worked, so he could confirm that this had been a mental problem all along.

To my neurologist, my belief that my physical symptoms constituted a physical problem was merely a symptom of mental distress. In 1951, American sociologist Talcott Parsons published *The Social System*, in which he coined the term *sick role*. Parsons asserted that when a person becomes ill—in any capacity, whether from the flu or permanent disability—they assume a role of "sanctioned deviance." That is, in addition to being physically ill, they adhere to a sick mindset that allows them to shirk social responsibilities and prevents them from wanting to get better. (This notion is particularly asinine in the United States, where one is entitled only to the health one can purchase and where poverty is enforced as a requirement for receiving disability benefits.) The sick role, according to Parsons, was intended to be a short-term social contract, and it was the duty of the medical establishment to police its abusers: patients who remained ill. Ideally, Parsons argued, diagnosis could be avoided altogether, as the sick role was "a mechanism which in the first instance channels deviance so that the two most dangerous potentialities, namely, group formation and successful establishment of the claim to legitimacy are avoided." Parsons was cited in social science research for decades before the theory of the sick role went out of favor in the 1990s. But this mode of thinking—with its fear of the articulatory capacity of diagnosis and its insistence upon work as a health outcome—has irreparably advanced the idea of the chronic illness patient as a malingerer who refuses to lay down their incapacitated life to the needs of the market.

An 1887 painting by André Brouillet called *A Clinical Lesson at the Salpêtrière* is the best-known visual rendering of hysteria. Before the viewer has time to analyze it, to speak of color or form or style, their gaze is drawn to Blanche Wittman, dipped back into a swoon, semiconscious and semi-undressed. She is hypnotized by Doctor Charcot, who is giving a medical demonstration to a window-lit audience of about thirty men. Many of whom, such as the neurologist Georges Gilles de la Tourette, can be identified by name and profession. Doc-

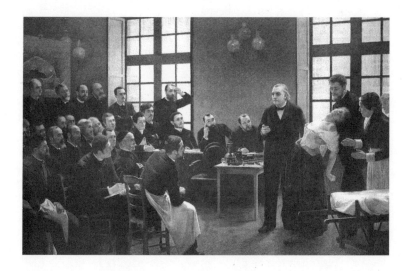

tors, artists, writers, and politicians attended Charcot's famed lectures, which served as the model for the modern teaching hospital. The scene depicted in the painting, appreciated by crowds at a salon hosted by the Académie des Beaux-Arts for its large canvas and overt sexuality, foretold the birth of psychoanalysis and expressed the spirit of neurology and psychology. In the painting, Charcot's gaze is out toward his audience: he is the only one not watching Blanche.

Professors Allan H. Ropper and Brian David Burrell write, "To understand this one painting is to understand everything that went wrong in the modern concept of mind and brain. It portrays nothing less than the original sin of neurology and psychiatry, one from which we are still trying to recover."

I spent the final stretch of high school sick, depressed, and underperforming in college acceptances. What I really wanted was to disappear entirely, but the concerned phone calls my school placed to my mother about my weight ensured that there would be no such reprieve granted to me. I went through the motions. I stopped wearing black, which I was told emphasized my pale complexion and made me look sickly. I studied makeup tutorials to learn how to appear more awake and alive, in a way I hoped was not obvious, because I believed that complicity in my own oppression was in poor taste. I clipped wefts of hair extensions onto my head to fill out my hair where illness and nutritional deficiencies had thinned it. I felt that if I didn't capture some image of health for myself, even one that was the result of concealed labor, I might soon be unable to conjure one. ("Everything in her," wrote Bourneville about Augustine, "announces the hysteric. The care that she takes in her toilette; the styling of her hair, the ribbons she likes to adorn herself with.") I did not keep many photos from that time, and my journal entries faded from a cacophony of questions, ideas, and quotes copied from novels to the occasional entry of symptoms. Graduating seniors were shown a video urging us to be vaccinated for meningitis, lest we perish to meningococcal disease in the college dorms; I remember thinking I already frequently experienced most of the symptoms of meningitis. I tried to escape the dullness of my destiny—an enduring illness and no reason to anticipate diagnosis; a declining ability to focus on reading, my life's other source of intensity since young childhood and the source of most of my knowledge about the world—by focusing on the experiences I believed to have been stolen from me that I might soon aggressively pursue: learning to cook, reading bad poetry, writing worse poetry, drinking all I could, falling in love with men and women, listening to Bach and Wagner as loud as I wanted without anyone to tell me to turn it down. I moved to an apartment, which was cheaper and quieter than a dorm. While the kind of romantic delusion I craved might make a fitting motivation for a fictional heroine, at university, I settled into life as a young woman in mourning for her body. My peers struck me as unromantic, utilitarian: eating, drinking, sleeping, fucking. In my eyes, they used their health for nothing. No one tried to do anything with unusual grace or rigor. I wondered if they could possibly understand what it was like to have the body as a vessel attacked by itself. *Attacked.* Writing the word feels false—or true only insofar as I can find no better alternative. Dualism plagues everything. Yet, I *did*, and do, feel isolated from my body, from my faculties—where is that "I" located? The self that observes its own illness for a prolonged period of time is vulnerable to that mind-body split. When I was able to think clearly, I felt that my body had betrayed me and was running the course of illness while my mind remained intact.

I had no desire to teach dance. It was too much a reminder of what I could no longer do, and I hated the children—their knobby knees and bad turnout, their lightness, the way they moved through the world expecting their lives to amount to more than accidents and unexplained events. I chose to try modeling, which struck me as more discreet than acting. In some ways, the casting process felt akin to the medical one. Girls would stand in a line of more than fifty before being called in, one by one, to walk the length of a runway in high heels before a casting director, who might or might not choose to examine the bound folio of the girl's previous work: digital headshots, torn-out magazine pages, commercial stills, over-exposed high-flash runway shots by party photographers; her clothing size and bust, waist, and hip measurements on a card. The director usually took simple digital photos of us holding a sheet of printer paper featuring our name and agency and might ask for some very basic biographical information. The entire process took only a few minutes. All that mattered was how you showed up in the photos and if you'd fit in the clothes. A casting only occasionally yielded a job. The pay was usually pitiful and seemed inversely correlated with the perceived prestige. Each time I booked a stint modeling clothing that cost many thousands of dollars more than I would be paid, I wondered about the extent to which my success had come from my inability to keep food down. My agent told me that whatever I was doing was working and not to change a goddamn thing. I told her not to worry: There was nothing I *could* change. I would continue to look, by the industry standard of heroin chic from back in the 1990s, quite all right.

I wondered if Augustine ever got to see her images, if she was able to practice, make adjustments, before she once again stepped in front of the camera to return to herself—if she considered herself to be making a record or a portfolio, like our modeling books. Or—as her body was never photographed straight on, except when she was in a state of hypnosis—was she unrecognizable to herself? Did it seem that it was some other patient, or a dead relative, looking back at her? Maybe she experienced her photographs as an argument, as I did: *No, those are *my* eyes. *My* sinking cheekbones. She must have known that to be the star hysteric of the hospital, she didn't actually need to be the most beautiful or photogenic or charismatic, but rather, a blank slate to invite projection. *You can see *more*, I'd repeat to myself in the makeup artist's chair, like a chant. *You can see *more through less of me.* A skinny girl on a runway is really just a clothes hanger; a skinny girl in a print ad is a nothingness onto which the client can project any image, and it will appear cohesive, logical. Any rupture or return of myself threatened that cohesion: at a runway show in the cathedral turned event venue downtown, sold by the diocese after the 1994 earthquake, I was queasy and could not think of all the Communions—breaking, eating the body—that had happened there. The walls were still lined with confessionals; sloppy drunks pawed at one another, stumbled in and out. I was fitted into a cocktail dress in the former priest's quarters, a room nestled behind the altar. A drop of blood formed by a pin prick on my back; a red cocktail was thrust into my hand; lines of cocaine were passed around on an iPhone screen, a rare gesture of sisterhood among models. Were the women of the

Salpêtrière competitive, or did they find solace in their shared community? There is so little documentation of the hysterics' relationships with one another, and they seem to pose alone. In any case, we models needed to sufficiently loosen ourselves before making the viscous, Clydesdale walk down the runway and vanishing into the whiteness of the flashbulb. Did Augustine have something—a thimble of wine, maybe—that would allow her to assemble her gestures, take in the scene, arrange her outfit? Could she see her reflection in a mirror before being photographed? In an engraving of the hospital's photographic setup in *La Nature* in 1883, the subject sits upon a solitary bed in a sparsely furnished room gazing at the man who is operating the camera—he does not appear to be visually taking an account of her at all. How did Augustine turn these things into a single image that is not the darkroom and the hospital gown and the lighting but, somehow, the effigy of a sick girl? Did she need to make this visual catalogue to contain her symptoms in order to overcome the shame, the boredom of talking about herself?

Perhaps there was nothing Augustine could change about herself; she was doomed to recidivism, eternally returning to the studio in order to take her symptoms, her wayward body, her humiliation, her powerlessness, and mold them into a shape of her own. Or perhaps Charcot told her not to change a goddamn thing, and she was left with the same understanding I was now arriving at: that our bodies are objects managed by forces much larger than ourselves.

Things got worse when I started to smell things. Something burning in the middle of the night, coming from nowhere.

Rotting meat, from inside me. I wondered if anyone else could smell me, if I was decaying, dead on earth. I would make a cup of tea, light a candle, take a Xanax. In the night, I smelled burning flesh (though I had no reason to know what burning human flesh might smell like) and woke up in fevered sweats. I began to divide my symptoms into two categories: things I would tell a doctor and things I would not.

Writing, I decided, was something I could do without a face. The kind of bold certainty with which I approached my intelligence and my ability looks shockingly entitled in hindsight, but it was also the first practical decision I'd made for myself. One can write from bed.

Most mornings, I have a painkiller before coffee. Others, I can't get out of bed. In some ways, I have already fulfilled my fear of becoming that Balanchine teacher with the cultish glaze in her eye. I just skipped the career, the glory days.

It must have been apparent to Charcot, from the moment she arrived in the hysteria ward at the Salpêtrière, that Augustine would be his next medical celebrity. She is all symptom, or the idea of the symptom. She is a beautiful object of desire, a victim of misogyny, a Bartleby, a mascot, whatever you would like her to be. There isn't even historical consensus about what she called herself or what others called her. In nineteenth-century materials, she is never called Augustine; she is either X.L., L., X., Gl., Louise, Louise Gl., Louise Gleiz. or Louise Glaiz., or G. The first mention of "Augustine" I have found is in the second volume of the *Iconographie photographique de la Salpêtrière*, a landmark publication of medical photography that sought to present photographs as pure signs of a depicted patient's illness, clinical features divested of any interiority— it cannot be overemphasized that everything we might find beautiful or interesting in the images, all of the inflections of Augustine's bodymind, exist despite the manner in which they were captured and recorded. The first edition includes no captions or case histories to describe the photographs, only section titles that categorize the patients as hysterics, epileptics, or "varia"—miscellaneous. After the second volume of the photographs from the Salpêtrière was released in 1878, a reviewer from the *British Medical Journal* griped, "We must say that we regret the work of such great scientific interest should be to English readers rendered somewhat unsavoury reading by the introduction of long pages of the obscene ravings of delirious hysterical girls, and descriptions of their sexual history . . . if described in the loose words of the patient when delirious and completely under the influence of a hystero-epileptic attack, such description may be interesting to the inquisitive student of disease and human nature, but is actually, in the words of the law-courts, 'matter unfit for publication.'"

My study of Augustine is often enveloped in the wordless color and texture of a Balanchine ballet or thick brain fog. I wonder if her story and mine are doomed to remain primarily imagistic. The fundamental unease of observing the photographs of the Salpêtrière patients so easily gives way to a bitter delight in an environment where normative, idealized bodies are understood to have gone wrong. Whether or not she was conscious, or had intent, or got to see her images, it is Augustine's relationship to her own body and her own image that holds my captivation. I am skeptical of the purported cultural value in allowing oneself to be visually documented; when I observe the images taken of me in my modeling years, I see not feminist tools of resistance, but a woman ambushed by economic necessity into an unsavory state of self-corroboration. In those photos, I am cold, bereft, absent; aligned with the aesthetic of the time but also characteristically withholding, austere.

At the Salpêtrière, a hysteric's symptoms were recognized only when they presented in visual form. In her photographs—I have come to think of them as fundamentally hers—Augus-

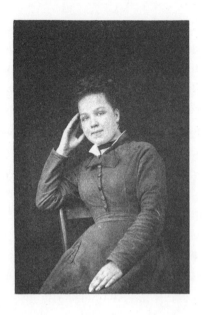

tine expresses one big emotion at a time. Joy. Confusion. Pain. Fear. The most neutral is the first photo, taken of her after her arrival, when she was about fourteen. "Normal State" features her sitting calmly, upright, in civilian clothes, comfortably poised in front of the camera, her gaze meeting it directly. Her cheekbones are high, her features symmetrical, and she is unashamed and wearing a slight smile. There is nothing of hysteria in the image. Though eighteen pages of notes follow, covering twenty-one months of her life and many more dramatic gestures, tics, and grimaces—allegedly in correlation with corporeal pathologies—next to nothing can be learned about her life from the volumes documenting her symptoms. Nevertheless, Paul Regnard, who took the medical photographs, knew something about capturing a woman. Augustine is always perfectly lit, well framed, and you can tell she has color in her face, which was something I envied.

My symptoms eventually kept me from sleeping even when my lifestyle didn't; everything had fallen apart with several agents, and everything showed in the camera. Augustine is never swallowed up by the light of the camera the way I was and must have practiced holding the passionate poses for a great deal of time. Despite having been subjected to medical tests in which doctors "pulled her hair, tickled, punched, and pricked her; they examined the mucous membranes of her eyelids, nostrils, mouth, tongue, and vulva . . . tested her hearing, vision, taste, and sense of smell," in the photos, she always appears untouched, distant, possessed only by herself and the singular emotion overtaking her, labeled clearly under each photo. It is never apparent what the depicted medical symptom *is*, other than a feeling. Augustine was received in the same manner as the pathologized ballet-girl who had preceded her by three decades, and by she who lived 125 years after.

The Salpêtrière women's costumes differ dramatically to convey something about their state. Fashion historian Yaara Keydar writes, "Before the[ir] attacks, the women are seen fully dressed in tight, tailored dresses, with a tight corset easily recognizable by the silhouette, their waistline emphasized and their hair worn up. In photographs taken during their attacks, however, they are shown wearing white, sheer gowns, stretching in different positions in bed, their hair loose and the curves of their bodies easily discernible." As writer Maayan Goldman puts it, "Both in the admission reports and in these black and white photographs, we are almost made to believe that the madwoman

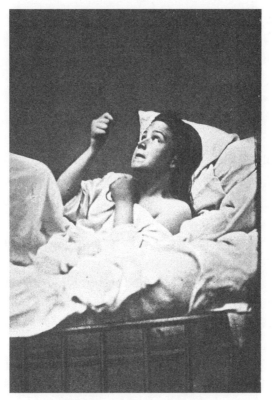

Passionate Attitudes: Menace

aesthetic is what's revealed underneath women's proper clothes once we 'peel' fashion's skin off." A woman's performance—her ability to mimic symptoms while under hypnosis, clad in a sartorial code used to signify her state of health or distress—could be read as a ratification of disease.

Charcot decided that "grand hysteria," or major hysteria, was characterized by episodic convulsions and four distinct, isolated phases: First, there is the epileptoid phase of seizures, preceded by an aura: a warning state in which changes in brain activity yield symptoms like visual disturbances, unusual smells or tastes, numbness, or tingling. (An image of Augustine in bed wearing her hospital gown, her mouth open and her tongue sticking out. Leather straps hold her to the bed. The photograph is labeled "Onset of the Attack: Cry.") Second, there are grand movements and contortions, like the famous hyperextended arch of the back. The third and most captured phase was the *attitudes passionnelles*, or "passionate poses," during which the patient acted out emotional gestures: ecstasy, eroticism, auditory hallucination, amorous supplication, menace, mockery. Finally, the fourth phase, delirium.

What can this tell us about illness or diagnosis? Probably very little. Sick girls often have to learn to pose, perhaps.

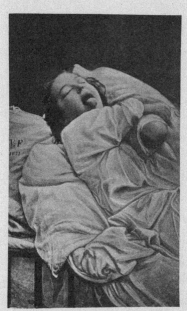

Planche XXVIII.

DÉBUT D'UNE ATTAQUE

CRI

Stéphane Mallarmé, who watched an astounding amount of ballet and theater despite finding most of it unbearably banal, attended the theater in search of an elusive *idée*, some invisible divine presence transcending whatever was happening on the stage, something free of representation and shallow spectacle. His poet's eye, as he describes it in the prose poem "Un spectacle interrompu," allows the poet to see more than what is visible, prioritizing intellectual or imaginative elements—insight rather than sight. It makes sense, then, that he was more moved by the abstract, theatrically lit dances of Loie Fuller than any romantic story ballet: "Here brought to Ballet is the atmosphere, or nothing," the "nothing" here being the elusive divine spirit of man, free from representation. Transcendent nothingness may have been Mallarmé's object of admiration, but in her famous Serpentine Dance, Fuller was likely imitating the hysterics. In her memoir, *Fifteen Years of a Dancer's Life*, she describes the takeoff of her career after performing the dance, which was based on a medical parody play, *Quack, M.D.*, noting that "hypnotism at that moment was very much to the fore in New York." The play features a scene of "hypnotic suggestion" from Dr. Quack: "I endeavoured to make myself as light as possible, in order to give the impression of a fluttering figure obedient to the doctor's orders. He raised his arms. I raised mine. Under the influence of suggestion, entranced—so, at least, it looked—with my gaze held by his, I followed his every motion."

In *Dance Pathologies*, McCarren articulates early modern dances like Fuller's as a response to the tradition of dance's resemblance to hysteric poses. She writes, "Mallarmé's dance texts on Loie Fuller record a shift away from the spectacular and toward the specular as Fuller's dance offers its spectators not simply sight, but insight." On Fuller's subsequent dances, which incorporated the theatrical lighting for which she came to be known, "Mallarmé describes [her] performing persona as facilitated by the 'absolute gaze' created by elec-

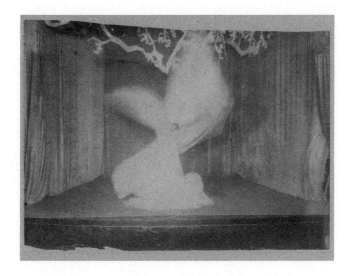

tric light, a gaze that can be identified with what Foucault refers to as the 'absolute gaze' of the nineteenth-century physician newly armed with instruments." The dancer under the absolute gaze is hypnotized, electrified, but the distinction of Fuller, Mallarmé says, is that she is self-hypnotized; her electric lighting is of her own creation. Her "use of the clinical apparatus used to diagnose and treat hysteria," McCarren says, "functions as a critique of Charcotian psychology, and reveals to what extent technological agency imposes a hierarchy of well and ill."

Once, in college, I decided to give modern dance a try, to see if that which was less physically demanding on my body might provide abstract, imaginative insight to me, too. The student choreographer explained that she saw each of our roles as representing one of the mental illnesses portrayed in the movie adaptation of Susanna Kaysen's *Girl, Interrupted*, a memoir of time spent in an institution following a suicide attempt. We were to portray a schizophrenic, a pathological liar, a woman with OCD, and a sociopath. I was assigned Kaysen's own borderline personality disorder. For the performance, we were to wear hospital gowns the color of Easter eggs. I dropped out of the production, popped a Vicodin, and went to a ballet class.

At Gucci's spring/summer 2020 show in Milan, the luxury brand stirred up controversy with models wearing straitjackets and institutional uniforms ferried down a conveyor belt in a clinical white room. One model held up her hands in silent protest, the words "Mental Health Is Not Fashion" scrawled in black marker across her palms. The message, however well-meaning, is untrue. Fashion doesn't really start trends; it condenses and visualizes something already around us. Runway shows rely on metaphor, grasping at the most suitable euphemisms for the anxieties of the time: wearable technology prods at the surveillance state; Balenciaga and Vetements's references to eastern Europe's 1990s affinity for American exports expresses neoliberal despair; Viktor and Rolf's meme gowns (SORRY I'M LATE I DIDN'T WANT TO COME; I'M NOT SHY I JUST DON'T LIKE YOU) highlight the poisoning of a terminally online generation. Anything can be fashion. As such, clothing has represented concerns about mental health, illness, pain, incarceration, and the medical gaze for longer than runways have existed. There's the *pouf à l'inoculation*, a woman's headdress created in support of inoculation against smallpox in the 1770s. Marie Antoinette's use of the pouf, which featured symbols of strength, peace, and medicine, helped popularize inoculation. Late eighteenth-century women gestured homage to guillotine victims of the French Revolution by wearing ribbons and chokers around their necks. Victorians romanticized the pale, emaciated figure withering from tuberculosis, which recurred with the "heroin chic" looks of the 1990s. In present-day Japan, the *yami-kawaii* (sick-cute) look, which emerged from online subcultures, uses sickly pale skin, red puffy eyes, and accessories of fake guns, syringes, gas masks, pills, and bandages to achieve a fragile, ill aesthetic—often considered a response to stigma surrounding mental health or to the psychological duress of the country's 2011 earthquake, tsunami, and nuclear meltdown. Gucci's straitjackets weren't even very original by contemporary standards. Alexander McQueen's spring/summer 2001 show featured models walking through a clinical glass box that turned into white padded cells adorned with surveillance mirrors that allowed the audience to watch the models, though the models could not see the audience. Before they made their entrance, McQueen reportedly told the models, "I need you to go mental." In the Regency period, many people were very concerned with the effects of thin or revealing clothing on their health. Thin muslin dresses left women cold and susceptible to illness, or "muslin disease"—though it is not clear if this term was actually used in the rhetoric of the era. The earliest reference I've found, thanks to an admirably unyielding dress historian on Twitter, is in an 1807 Munich journal: "A doctor in Northern Germany warns against a new disease which, in varying forms, threatens the fair sex with death and doom; he calls it the muslin disease."

According to Gucci, the spring/summer 2020 show's controversial opening looks were not intended to be sold. They were the "most extreme version of a uniform dictated by society and those who control it." Creative director Alessandro Michele designed "these blank-styled clothes to represent how, through fashion, power is exercised over life." To be generous, Gucci's straitjackets are in conversation with fashion's long-standing representations of "madness." The straitjacket obstructs our true—perhaps mad—nature, whereas the subsequent looks in Gucci's collection purportedly allow our nature to break free. Fashion is positioned as the antidote to restraint, enabling expression through clothes and accessories. None of this, of course, is "political." This fantasy ethos of the fashion industry is poorly positioned to meaningfully represent the subjectivity of a sick person. And yet the use of "sick" imagery suggests a fixation on illness and pain. A runway show, when best executed and carried to its logical conclusion, acts as a pathography. Even so, fashion is seldom revelatory. Slippery metaphors and vague references reign.

Susan Sontag saw that only a certain kind of pain image makes its way into Western art history: "The sufferings most often deemed worthy of representation are those understood to be the product of wrath, divine or human. (Suffering from natural causes, such as illness or childbirth, is scantily represented in the history of art; that caused by accident, virtually not at all—as if there were no such thing as suffering by inadvertence or misadventure.)"

Although tuberculosis was a popular motif in painting, chronic pain and prolonged illness are rare subjects for visual

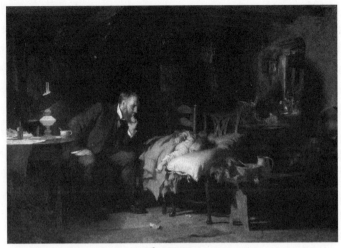

The Doctor

art. When you find them, they are often deathbed scenes and say more about those gathered in the final moments than about the suffering itself. Many such works do not foreground the body of the sick person: Luke Fildes's 1891 painting, *The Doctor*, commissioned as a work of social realism, depicts a pensive doctor watching over a child patient, whose face is partially obstructed by a tuft of hair. In 1947, the painting was featured on a US Postal Service stamp for the centenary of the American Medical Association. Two years later, the AMA used the image in its campaign against nationalized medical care as proposed by President Truman: emblazoned across posters and brochures, instructing the reader to "Keep Politics Out of This Picture." Contrastingly, in Britain, the painting was used as an emblem of celebration for the National Health Service.

In Edvard Munch's 1896 work, *By the Deathbed (Fever)*, the face of the sick person is again obstructed. The title subject in the series of six paintings called *The Sick Child*, based on Munch's sister, dead of tuberculosis at age fifteen, is blurred, shown in profile, staring past a doting, grieving figure toward a dark, ominous curtain. Though the series is often lauded as "a vivid study of the ravages of a degenerative disease," it isn't apparent whether there is anything degenerative about the child's condition: propped up against a large pillow, she holds the hand of her caretaker, who appears to offer her some small comfort in light of her waning time. In a subsequent painting, *Death in the Sickroom*, Munch shifts the focus farther from the girl's physical state: As she sits in a chair facing a corner of the room, she appears partially transparent. The mourners who gather around her retreat into themselves, unsure of how to address or account for the girl, who is withering away before their eyes. The scene doesn't quite depict empathy, but what it shows is preferable to pity. The sick subject is rarely *the* subject. I cannot recall seeing a painting from the point of view of the person convalescing in a sickbed or emergency room or trying to write in the midst of pain-induced brain fog.

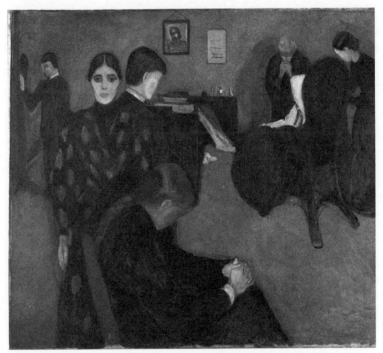

Death in the Sickroom

Why do I retain attachment to such a famously problematic word, *hysteria*, when it invites metaphor and messy historical analogy? Rachel Mesch writes that the contemporary feminist answer to the question of hysteria can be summarized through two broad directions:

> [The first] examines the gender hierarchy of the medical profession and its victimization of women through history and literature; in this light, the hysteria diagnosis is revealed to have unfairly silenced women who threatened the social order. The other trend takes a more psychoanalytic perspective, seeing hysteria, in Carol Smith-Rosenberg's terms, as a desperate "flight into illness." From this perspective radical French feminists like Hélène Cixous, Catherine Clément, and Luce Irigaray recognize hysteria as a form of female resistance. Irigaray, for example, recognizes the revolutionary potential of the hysteric as a "culturally induced symptom." Irigaray's hysteric herself deliberately assumes the feminine role, carrying on a charade of feminized suffering to, in her words "convert a form of subordination into an affirmation, and thus begin to thwart it."

In everyday use, *hysteria* still means "uncontrolled or dramatic emotional display," but in the Lacanian psychoanalysis clinic, the hysteric holds revolutionary potential. It was Lacan who, in his four discourses, set up the hysteric's discourse as that which can overturn fixity and uncover new lines of inquiry. In a Lacanian clinic, a hysteric diagnosis is far from an affront: as the psychoanalyst Anouchka Grose puts it, "Dissatisfaction is the motor for desire, and desire drives existence. Hysterics specialise at using dissatisfaction to keep desire spinning, acting against atrophy and ossification. Far from trying to get them to stop fussing and get back in line, one might encourage them to take their questioning further, to use it in their lives and work, and to even attempt to enjoy it." If, as Lacan said, the only distinction between humans and animals is that we are afraid of our shit, the hysteric, unafraid of paradox or truth or shit, can be seen as a seeker, someone who uses her discomforts and dissatisfactions as means to interrogate the Other. The hysteric's dissatisfaction keeps desire spinning—a preferable interpretation to the body-as-contradiction being problematized.

One need not endorse Freud's theory of hysteria as unconscious ideas or desire that manifests itself in symptoms in order to use it toward an idea's shape. After reading Freud enthusiastically, the artist Louise Bourgeois entered analysis in 1952, at the age of forty. She was experiencing a cluster of symptoms (insomnia, depression, fits of anger, agoraphobia, dizziness, sore throats, nausea) and dichotomous digestive issues, many consistent with those previously attributed to hysteria. The emotional turmoil she experienced after the death of her father ("literally cannot live or function / without the protection of a father," reads a diary entry from 1952) encouraged her to seek treatment. Bourgeois's work invites psychoanalytic narrative as an entry point, returning again and again to a common family drama: her father was unfaithful to her invalid mother by sleeping with Louise's governess, and her mother tacitly used Louise to keep an eye on the affair. The story could have been adapted from any number of the case studies in Freud and Breuer's *Studies in Hysteria*. Bourgeois wrote, "Since the fears of the past were connected with the functions of the body, they reappear through the body. For me, sculpture is the body. My body is my sculpture." Much of her work seems to replicate Freud's structure of symptom formation, though *The Arch of Hysteria* maintains the most explicit dialogue: a hanging figure of a male body cast in bronze is bent backward in a maneuver reminiscent of the *arc-de-cercle*, a famed pose of the hysteria patients at the Salpêtrière in which the body is arched upward, locked in spasm, with weight only on the head and feet. In neither the case of the patients nor in Bourgeois's symbolic body is it clear if the body is in pain or pleasure, if it is expressing illness or jouissance—or, if illness, if it is caused by or reflects the mind. In both cases, the body is frozen, exposed, defenseless, suspended in time.

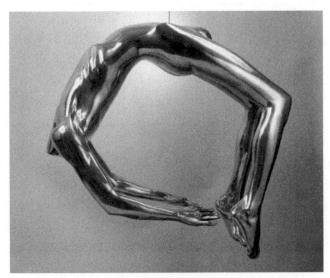

The Arch of Hysteria

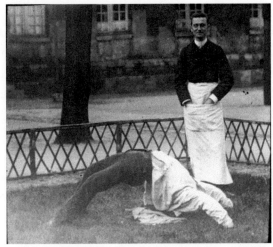

*A male Salpêtrière patient photographed by Albert
Londe sometime between 1859 and 1910*

Curator and writer Philip Larratt-Smith writes that Bourgeois was mistrustful of psychoanalysis's process of bringing the unconscious to light through dreams, slips of the tongue, and somatic symptoms and, instead, preferred to access her unconscious through sculpture—through the body: "In Bourgeois's terms, the successful realization of a sculpture functions to make conscious what was previously unconscious—that is, repressed and inaccessible—and to discharge unwelcome or unmanageable instinctual impulses."

Without dance to help me live, my symptoms continued to present as unwelcome, unmanageable impulses. I was accused, in equal measure, of dehumanizing pleasure-seeking and being too broken to have healthy desire. Desire, contained by bodily capability, was difficult to gauge. My body was cold, my appendages blue, my bedroom a mausoleum of pills and too-bright lights. How to warm myself, circulate blood? Sometimes the heat of sex seemed the only possible antidote, and my anguished desperation overwhelmed my companion. At other times, when a man crawled into my bed, I articulated my state in staccato gestures: the opiates on the nightstand, the eleventh hour on the clock, a new rash, the lack of sensation in my toes. I'd sense his disappointment, or his suspicion that this was all a product of vanity. I would feel his interest lift like a fog—for me, a relief.

Bourgeois frequently wrote of her inability to make herself loved and of her struggle to relate to men sexually and emotionally. She experienced herself as a void, one who existed as a woman only in relation to a man: "The empty house / means that I am identified with / the void, it isn't out there any longer / I am the void." Psychoanalyst Juliet Mitchell writes, "Bourgeois shows that what psychoanalysis considers to be *inevitable* is, in fact, the *impossible* condition of a woman's sexuality within patriarchy."

My body continued to find new things intolerable. My beloved Mitsouko perfume suddenly produced migraines. The man who gave it to me had explained that scents could have narrative arcs, like ballets or novels. One of the first true chypres, the scent was based on Jacques Guerlain's love affair with Japanese culture—or perhaps with a woman he met in Japan—but there is nothing Japanese about Mitsouko aside from the name. Like the male protagonist in a Stravinsky ballet, Guerlain didn't know what he was talking about, the man had told me. Obviously, I did not call a doctor to complain about not being able to wear a perfume.

There's no such thing as an aesthetic illness, a boyfriend once said to me. *Do you even* want *to get better?*

Charcot was almost completely uninterested in his patients' words, even when they were reenacting traumatic, often sexual episodes—Augustine's visions included "rape, blood, more fires, terrors, and hatred of men"; scenes from novels she had read; and, according to Bourneville, the hallucination that "when the men around her speak, flames emerge from their mouths." It is difficult to imagine, given the pointed nature of the hallucinations, but Charcot considered anything said during a hysteric attack to be "vocalization, not communication, a clinical feature that helped to differentiate hysteria from diseases it resembled, such as epilepsy." During one of his lectures, he presented to his viewers a hysteric in the midst of an attack. She called out, "Mama, I'm scared," after which, Charcot remarked to his audience, "You see how hysterics scream. One could say that is a lot of noise about nothing. Epilepsy is more serious and much more silent." But Augustine was a talkative girl. During another demonstration, Charcot induced a contraction of her tongue and larynx muscles, leaving her mute for six days.

Sometimes, Augustine relived traumatic incidents from her childhood through her attacks. She'd been sent to a convent school in a small town forty miles east of Paris at age six, where she remained until she was thirteen. She relished long walks in the countryside there, during which she befriended an older woman stuck in a miserable marriage with an abusive husband—when she was ten, the man turned his attention to Augustine, and attempted to sexually assault her. Her most potent memory, which she frequently acted out during attacks, was of a man she called Mr. C. Augustine was sent to Mr. C.'s household to work as a servant when she was thirteen. He brutally assaulted her, and six days later, Augustine had her first attack of hysteria while gazing into the eyes of a cat. Daily attacks followed, which were addressed, unsuccessfully, with bloodletting. Augustine suffered her most intense attack after running into Mr. C. while doing an errand. The scenes following Mr. C.'s assault on her foretold why observations of hysterics would later serve as the basis for psychoanalysis. While her attacks became milder once she was working as a chambermaid for an elderly woman, she also developed an interest in two of her brothers' friends and became sexually active with each of them. When her parents found out, they were furious, and in the midst of that fury, family confidences were revealed: Augustine learned that her father believed that her brother was not his son and that her mother had been sleeping with Mr. C. Asti Hustvedt notes, "While it is not mentioned in the text, this revelation raises the real possibility that her brother is her rapist's son. Augustine also finds out that her mother had sold her daughter to Mr. C. as a sexual favor." The structure of the episode alludes to Freud's case study of Dora—who was implicitly handed over by her father to his lover's husband to fulfill the cost of his adultery—and to countless others in *Studies in Hysteria*.

Augustine would see Mr. C. one more time, when he came to the Salpêtrière for one of Charcot's lectures, presumably with the hope of catching a glimpse of the young woman he had assaulted. "A man like you, a forty-year-old man," Augustine recounted to Bourneville, while she was possibly in a hallucinatory state, "what do you know about medicine . . . You will not see me in the class . . . I have decided to tell . . . On two Sundays . . . Why did I hide my face in the class . . . Because of you."

While Charcot sought to identify an organic biological illness causing the hysterics' symptoms, Bourneville was more inclined toward considering the psychological context of the patients. He paid attention to the consistency of trauma in the histories of the women of the Salpêtrière years before Freud developed methods to force them to relive it, repeatedly, in the hope that something useful might emerge. Bourneville justified including a great deal of information about each patient's life, "so that our readers can clearly appreciate the different phases of the delirium phase of the attack." It was with Bourneville that Augustine felt she could speak and be heard. It was Bourneville's idea to photograph the hysteria patients in Charcot's ward, to allow them to speak through, or be lost in, the language of images.

Why does talking about trauma remain one of the only socially acceptable ways women can discuss health, discomfort, or pain? I would like to prize my object of reflection over my feelings about it, but in the limbo of medical illegibility, the object is reduced to the feeling.

I saw more doctors, tried to answer more devastating, hopeless questions. Had I ever had joint stiffness in the morning, for at least an hour, lasting for more than six weeks? (Yes.) Had I noticed nodules under the skin around my ankles and elbows? (Yes.) Erythema nodosum, tender, red bumps on the shins? (Yes.) Had I experienced night sweats? (Yes.) Jaw pain when chewing? (No.) Sudden, rapid hair loss? (Yes.) Amenorrhea? (Yes.) Had I experienced a gritty, sandy feeling in my eyes? (Yes.) Neck pain? (Yes.) Rashes on my cheeks? (Yes.) For more than a month? (No.) Psoriasis? (No.) Rashes (not sunburn) after sun exposure? (Yes.) Sores in the mouth or nose for more than two weeks at a time? (Yes.) Dry mouth? (Yes.) Fingers unusually sensitive to cold? (Yes.) Fingers changing color in the cold? (Yes.) Blood clots in lungs or legs? (No.) Angina? (No.) Chest pain made worse by breathing and lasting for more than a few days? (No.) Asthma? (Yes.) Had I ever had tuberculosis? (No.) Frequent abdominal pain? (Yes.) Blood in stool? (Yes.) Nausea?

(Yes.) Heartburn? (Yes.) Muscle weakness for more than three months? (Yes.) Muscle cramps? (Yes.) Weakness or dizziness when rising from a sitting position lasting for more than three months? (Yes.) Neurologic numbness or tingling? (Yes.) Pulmonary fibrosis? (No.) Thyroid disease? (No.) Lymphoma? (No.) Easy bruising? (Yes.) Swollen lymph nodes? (Yes.) Hives? (Yes.) Eczema? (Yes.) Pain with urination? (Yes, from frequent bladder infections.) Ulcers on vagina, penis, or scrotum? (Yes, but with negative STD tests.) Infertility? (Almost certainly.) Miscarriage? (No.) Depression? (Ha!)

"He used to look again and again at things he did not understand," Freud wrote of Charcot, "to deepen his impression of them day by day, till suddenly an understanding of them dawned on him." Charcot, the great visual observer. Freud's revolutionary contribution was to see the hysteria patients as speaking subjects. Symptoms that could previously be interpreted only through their visual presentation could now be spoken about, be interpreted through language. Freud's interpretation of hysteria symptoms as "compromise formations" created by the collision of the repressed idea or desire with the suppression, hybridizes them: the symptom is both articulated and repressed, both psychic and embodied.

It was only by chance that my unchanging bodily situation acquired a name. A doctor—perhaps in acquiescence to my pleading, but probably not—made a new suggestion: *Write down what happened.* A short history, listing my symptoms, when pain began, and how it progressed. *Write down how you feel each day. We'll see if it adds up to anything.* The instruction was likely a patronizing acquiescence to my clarion distress as opposed to a genuine attempt to obtain information that could be useful for my treatment. Yet, I found the potential gravity of the task comforting: When you point out that something has been taken for granted, it is about to be so no longer. I searched for edges, in order to give what I had gone through some recognizable form so it could be acknowledged, acted upon. How I was *then* versus *now.* When did the pain become regular? Has it been a week? A month? A year? The more I thought about when I might have last been healthy, the more a figure of "a self with health" was formed in my mind. My penmanship—which, in the days before the arthritis really took hold, was quite neat—in these entries appears frenzied, trembling, as though every cell in my body were popping with effervescence, irrepressible. The more I wrote down for the doctor, the more pain I found already there in the darkness, outside myself, tenses tangled. I could be fresh, new in each moment of observation. When I wrote about an ache lifting, I was euphoric—*the pills must be helping!* Reading the notes now, I bore myself. The writing's relentless self-awareness does not excuse its ragged edges, its intrusive mediocrity. The self-fascination seemingly required to own one's *I* is my ultimate reservation: one's own pain is simply not a tasteful object of contemplation. Yet, the *I* ideally contains fragments, inconsistencies, that might prove to be fruitful, allow me to exist within the experience, avoid re-narrativizing the past.

The doctor had told me to write down the facts, but the facts . . . *weren't*, exactly. My symptoms were as they always were: *fever; dizzy all the time; things sound different than usual, echo-y.* Each felt like a climax, but only the fever could be turned into data, could transform the unruly events of the body into information. *I am trying to cultivate a way of being that will keep me from being swallowed by time spent like this, with no end in sight.* Sentence accomplished. *But to accept living this way would be a violation of my life.* I believed that writing what I experienced—even through some unwritten omission—might bring a useful interpretation to the surface, or that a hidden logic between ostensibly disconnected symptoms and ideas would reveal itself.

In Agnes Varda's 1962 film *Cléo from 5 to 7*, a pop singer receives an omen of death in a fortune-teller's tarot card reading. The film follows Cléo for the next two hours as she awaits the results of a biopsy that could reveal cancer. During this time, she moves through the world as someone who is both sick and healthy. Her assistant, lover, and fellow musicians—whose attention Cléo courts and deflects—dismiss her fear, call her a hypochondriac, and ridicule her for worrying about something they believe to be psychosomatic, echoing the common cultural perception of the era that cancer was a disease caused or exacerbated by anxiety and repression. To those around her, Cléo is not sick; and if she is, she herself is at fault, as the illness is a result of her having let unfavorable aspects of her personality flourish. The film is especially potent in its exploration of the cultural charges placed on illness, particularly that which says illness makes someone more or less beautiful. In an inner monologue, Cléo reassures herself: "Ugliness is a kind of death. As long as I'm beautiful, I'm more alive than others." She tries on hats in a boutique and admires her reflection, even as pedestrians gaze at her through the shop window. What initially seems like vanity is revealed to be contemplation, as Cléo weighs what she believes has made her life up to this point valuable. The way she regards herself, in the face of the possibility of a life spent sick or of death, becomes the ultimate definer of how the world views her, too: At the beginning of the film, she steps into an intersection, confident that she will be able to stop traffic, which she does. Later, after her self-assurance is worn away from concern, she attempts to pass through a line of pedestrians, but no one moves; they don't even notice her.

Despite his effort to do so, Charcot never discovered any physical origin or organic cause for hysteria. I began to wonder which illnesses might have been considered to be hysteria during his reign at the Salpêtrière—certainly, if he had witnessed my fainting spells or convulsions, he might have diagnosed me a hysteric. Eventually, hysteria became an illness associated with the mind. It's often said that Charcot "invented" hysteria, meaning he coined the name for the collection of symptoms (including emotional excess, sexual desire, seizures, anxiety, and eating disorders) that occurred in a large number of women. The modern equivalents of the symptoms he observed at the Salpêtrière are thought to be functional illness, somatization disorder, or conversion disorders—Freud was the first to use the third term in 1893: "If, for the sake of brevity, we adopt the term 'conversion' to designate the transformation of psychical excitation into chronic somatic symptoms which distinguishes hysteria"—all of which lack clear clinical diagnostic criteria and are ascribed to women, like me, who have not yet been told what is wrong with them.

It's surprising—given the insistence of multiple neurologists that my fainting spells were the result of unrealized depression or anxiety—that I was never diagnosed with a conversion disorder. Today, conversion disorders are thought to be psychiatric, even when a neurological symptom like numbness, paralysis, blindness, seizures, deafness, or losing the ability to speak is present. These symptoms are thought to present after a trauma or psychological trigger, and the conversion disorder diagnosis is made after other possibilities are ruled out. It is curious that Charcot insisted on investigating hysteria as biological given his early use of the term *traumatic hysteria* to describe the psychopathological impact of train accidents on passengers. In 1898, a law was established, based on Charcot's science of *grand ébranlement psychique*, in order to compensate traumatized industrial workers who were the victims of accidents. French psychologist Pierre Janet agreed with Charcot that the onset of hysteria could begin with a shock, but he asserted that the *ideation* of a shock was enough for hysteria to take hold—for instance, in order for one's limb to become paralyzed, one need not be in an actual accident, but merely *imagine* an accident.

The contemporary conversion disorder isn't conceptually far from what Freud posited hysteria to be: somatic symptoms resulting from a psychic conflict. However, the *Diagnostic and Statistical Manual of Mental Disorders* preferences individual pathology, while Freud believed that hysteric symptoms emerged as unconscious protest against restrictive and patriarchal social conditions. It was Charcot's insistence upon examining hysteria in a purely biological framework that perpetuated a harmful paradigm; he asserted that women were somehow biologically prone to hysteria. As Jacqueline Rose puts it, "The problem with Charcot's work is that while he was constructing the symptomatology of the disease (turning it into a respected object of the medical institution), he was reinforcing it as a special category of behaviour, visible to the eye, and the result of a degenerate hereditary disposition." Freud intervened in order to challenge Charcot's visual evidence of hysteria and to deny hysteria as a distinct clinical entity. Hysteria's medicalization (the process by which something gets framed as principally a medical problem) focused on individual biological bodies under Charcot, on social conditions and trauma under Freud, and on individualized pathology devoid of consideration for systemic or infrastructural conditions by the most recent *DSM*.

Western medical discourse has never relinquished the insistence that an illness that can be observed in a scan or measured by a test is real and that one that cannot is likely unreal. In 2006, the *New York Times* ran an article titled "Is Hysteria Real? Brain Images Say Yes"—the troubling implication of the headline being that neurological or psychological disorders without observable brain qualities can be safely assumed to be "unreal." Of course, Salpêtrière hysteria patients' brains were not scanned; the article refers to conversion disorder patients in Western hospitals and equates the observation that the "emotional" structures of the brain could be moderating sensory and motor neural circuits with the disease's reality. Novelist Siri Hustvedt (sister of Asti) writes that the brain scans "demonstrate that there are neuroanatomical correlates to a hysterical paralysis or blindness—an organic change—but how that happens can't be discovered from an fMRI; nor do these images tell doctors how to treat their conversion patients."

Charcot never found his hysteria lesion. Some of my lesions eventually amounted to a diagnosis. While collecting a culture to confirm, once again, that the occasional lesions I had gotten since long before becoming sexually active were not, in fact, a sexually transmitted infection, my gynecologist said she was glad I had come in; she had been thinking of me. She had another patient, a young girl with the same lesions I had first experienced before puberty. The patient, apparently much more adept at navigating online symptom trackers than I was, sought out a rheumatologist, who used the lesions to diagnose her with a rare, congenital autoimmune disease of the blood vessels that caused myriad symptoms throughout the body's systems. Like me, this patient also experienced lesions in flares with other symptoms, had arthritis and fainting spells—due to swelling of the brain during episodes of blood vessel inflammation, she learned. Was it possible that I had the same illness?

Off I went to a rheumatologist. He said I was lucky to have the lesions, burning topical ulcers that were almost certainly indicative of Behçet's disease. Lesions meant a diagnosis, and a diagnosis is a gift. *Now*, he said to me, *we can know that all this suffering was not only in your head.*

The bad news was that little could be done, diagnosis was simply a confirmation of symptoms, which we would do our best to manage: oral ulcers; eye inflammation (possibly leading to blindness); rashes; genital sores; rheumatoid arthritis; swelling in the arms and legs; blood clots; digestive system upset, including abdominal pain, diarrhea, and bleeding; and inflammation of the brain and nervous system, causing headache, fever, disorientation, poor balance, or stroke. He took X-rays and pored over the slides with a red pen like a math teacher. He circled the places where my body could be more successful: the hyperextended joints that made my lines ideal for ballet were actually ill-suited for supporting the skeleton while performing daily activities and only worsened my symptoms of seronegative rheumatoid arthritis. I might sometimes "feel crazy" thanks to my occasionally swollen brain. My digestive tract is cratered with blisters. This is why "flavors" might hurt.

You're lucky, he said—repeating what people say when something terribly unlucky, something horrendous, has happened. *Many people with diseases like yours never find out what is wrong with them.*

He confirmed his diagnosis through a pathergy test: a small needle inserted into my forearm, where an irritated pustule would form a day later, indicating that my immune system was overreacting to a minor injury. I had observed my immune system overreacting to minor injuries my entire life—my bumps and bruises had always been resistant to healing, and I often formed lesions and rashes where they occurred—and had frequently described these observations to doctors. How could something so quaint be a diagnostic criterion?

On my way out, the rheumatologist offered me an antidepressant.

Looking at my medical records from those earlier years, it is difficult not to grow angry at the acutely deficient diagnostic process. Why, when I was growing up constantly sick and fevered, had my blood vitamin levels been checked but not the common inflammation markers associated with autoimmunity? Why had this also been the case in college, when I went to the hospital after fainting while sitting down? (*A rare occurrence*, I was told.) Why had it been that, the more I asked for what I knew I needed to survive (relief from pain, induced sleep in order to occasionally sleep through illness), the less it was offered to me? Why, when I relayed to a doctor that a massage therapist had told me I had Raynaud's—a condition resulting in decreased blood flow to the hands and feet, which is frequently predictive of other connective tissue disorders— had he done nothing to investigate further? Why had my growing medical articulateness been seen as inherently suspect? (*Do me a favor and stop reading about this*, one doctor had said when I brought to him papers on autoimmunity without the common biomarkers, which frequently go undetected. *It's no use*.) Why had I, an extremely active young person, been told that I could be as abled or disabled *as I wanted*, as if any of this had anything to do with what anyone wanted? Why had the gynecologist tasked with my annual exam—"Always the genital thing," Charcot reportedly said of hysteria to Freud, even as he investigated it as a disease of the nervous system— been the only one who took seriously the task of investigating symptoms ravaging other parts of my body? Why had it been easier for countless doctors over the course of more than a decade to chalk up the symptoms in *every bodily system* in my body to hysteria, when there wasn't even an agreement on what conversion disorders were, how they worked, or how they should be treated?

Behçet's, like many autoimmune diseases, is named after the doctor who first observed and classified it. Hulusi Behçet, a Turkish dermatologist, observed symptoms in a man from 1924 to 1925. Originally suspected to have syphilis or tuberculosis, the man completely lost his vision after several iridectomies to address his ocular inflammation. In 1930, Behçet saw a female patient with similar ocular irritation and with oral and genital ulcers; through biopsies, he ruled out syphilis, tuberculosis, and mycosis. In 1936, another, male patient showed the same symptoms, along with folliculitis, fevers in the evening, and abdominal pain. Behçet decided that these patients were sufficient in number for him to describe a new disease of inflamed blood vessels, and he published his findings. The disease remains rare in the United States and Europe but is endemic in East and Central Asia. My second rheumatologist, who asked if I was Turkish—I'm not—told me that someone in my family "might be lying about their ancestry."

Diagnosis of Behçet's is based on symptoms, as there is no test that conclusively detects the disease. Patients might live without diagnosis for many years because all their tests come back normal. When all your tests are normal, the verdict is usually that there is nothing wrong with you. With Behçet's, it is much easier to prove that there is nothing wrong with you than that there is something wrong with you. You will see a neurologist who will not detect a stroke or find a brain lesion, a gastroenterologist who will not detect Crohn's or IBS, a gynecologist who will not find any STDs, and so on. Yet, when all the symptoms are considered together, the range of possible causes narrows considerably. With Behçet's, we do not know the ultimate "cause" of the autoimmunity that impacts many bodily systems.

It is easier to research hysteria than Behçet's disease. The Los Angeles Public Library, where I discovered Augustine's photographs, houses only one book on my illness, published in 1997. The title assures me I am "not alone." A section on "preventive measures" in another Behçet's medical textbook suggests, "plenty of rest, maintain daily routine, reduce stress."

After years of her symptoms being written off as hysteria, Alice James was diagnosed with late-stage breast cancer in 1891. In her diary, she cuts to the heart of the self-understanding offered by the diagnosis:

> Ever since I have been ill, I have longed and longed for some palpable disease, no matter how conventionally dreadful a label it might have, but I was always driven back to stagger alone under the monstrous mass of subjective sensations, which that sympathetic being "the medical man" had no higher inspiration than to assure me I was personally responsible for, washing his hands of me with a graceful complacency under my very nose. Dr. Torry was the only

man who ever treated me like a rational being, who did not
assume, because I was victim to many pains, that I was, of
necessity, an arrested mental development too.

James suffered for most of her life, but it took cancer for her
symptoms to be treated as real. The epidemic of autoimmune
disease—chronic Lyme disease; myalgic encephalomyelitis/
chronic fatigue syndrome, or ME/CFS; fibromyalgia; long
Covid-19; and other poorly understood immune and nervous
system disorders—resides along a more complicated spectrum
from belief to cultural marginalization. I do, in some sense,
feel lucky to have been diagnosed with a condition with biomarkers and observable physical symptoms—as opposed to a
less visible condition that would have been received with even
greater medical skepticism or would continue to be treated
as an expression of underlying mental illness. Nevertheless, it
is difficult to view diagnosis as a "gift" when my illness keeps
me from living normally, speaking normally, eating normally,
sleeping normally, moving normally, writing normally. Diagnosis has changed nothing about my bodily situation except
what I am told I must endure in order to account for it. Because
there are no drugs developed specifically for Behçet's patients,
I am assigned medications intended to address gout and psoriasis. When I have a flare, I suppress it with steroids. Muscle
relaxers and antiepileptic drugs help me sleep. I implore a
rheumatologist to allow me to try *something, anything* but the
immune suppressants that make me even more susceptible to
infection, inviting in never-ending flu viruses and chronic uri-
nary tract infections. A new drug drastically improves my oral

ulcers (one of my most frequent symptoms), but destroys my hard-earned relationship with food: "Flavors" hurt worse than ever before. The smell of eggs in the morning makes me vomit.

A synthetic opiate helped my pain considerably but ushered in additional brain fog, alarming my pharmacist, who had been filling these same prescriptions for many years. She cited her concern that I'd been prescribed an "evil triad" of drugs, all ripe for addiction (I was given Tramadol, the muscle relaxer, and a low dose of Xanax, a prescription left over from the earlier days of my illness, when what I had was thought to be nothing but anxiety).

You're too young for all this, she told me, and refused to fill the prescriptions, even after my rheumatologist explained that I suffered from a rare disease that warranted them. (I know women whose prescriptions for miscarriage induction were refused by pharmacists, and trans people who were denied their hormones—presumably both due to religious moral objection, which, outrageously, is legal in the United States today—but I had no idea that pharmacists in California could override a doctor's orders and refuse to fill a prescription based on their own professional opinion of how a disease should be treated.) Now I fill my prescriptions at different pharmacies—a behavior associated with risky drug use. Even when a patient is "lucky" enough to have a condition with a "legitimate" diagnosis and has a job or resources that allow access to a medical specialist to advise treatment, there are endless opportunities for someone not living in their body to know better, to deny care, to make things more difficult, to tell the patient what they ought to do instead. All this because I learned the name of my disease.

In her memoir on her treatment for breast cancer, Anne Boyer writes, "Diagnosis has diminished my ability to tell the difference between good and empty ideology. Everything I am advised to do in response to the cancer seems, at first, like a symptom of a world that is sick itself."

Boyer alerts us to the dizzying impossibility not only of navigating what we "must" do to account for our illness, but also of the project of making literature about illness. So many accounts begin with a lament that there are no good books written on illness, that the experience of illness is resistant to or destructive of narrative. Virginia Woolf wondered why illness was never established as a serious project in literature; why the sick were, by default, outsiders who needed "a new language, more primitive, more sensual, more obscene." Readers, she suspected, might complain that illness "lacked plot." (I will not get better; nor am I likely to die anytime soon. My sense of possibility for my life diminishes with time lived.) Even in her essay on illness, Woolf only hints at the ailments that plagued her throughout her life, asserting that, in the matter of disease, "we go alone, and like it better so. Always to have sympathy . . . would be intolerable." Though she potently explores states of illness in her fiction—Rachel's delirious, raging fever in *The Voyage Out*; Rhoda's madness in *The Waves*; and Septimus's suicidal mania in *Mrs. Dalloway*—when she describes pain specifically her own, language does appear to have run dry. A biographer notes the pause Woolf's illness created in her work. Leonard was the documentarian of Virginia's illness.

Ever since American essayist Elaine Scarry asserted in 1985 that pain is unshareable and destroys language, inexpressibility has dominated the discourse to an even greater extent. Why bother, then? Why try to describe something that evades description, destroys language? Boyer rages against this, too: "Suppose for a moment the claims about pain's ineffability are historically specific and ideological, that pain is widely declared inarticulate for the reason that we are not supposed to share a language for how we really feel." Responding to Hannah Arendt's description of pain in *The Human Condition* as "the most private and least communicable" of all experience, Boyer continues:

> Contrast this philosophical truism about pain's lack of communicability with your own experience of witnessing another living creature in pain. The howls, cries, screams, shrieks, and whimpers of another in pain are unequivocal . . . The look of a face in pain—even a nonhuman face—cannot be mistaken for a look of contentment . . . Pain, indeed, is a condition that creates *excessive* appearance. Pain is a fluorescent feeling. That pain is incommunicable is a lie in the face of the near-constant, trans-species, and universal communicability of pain. So, the question, finally, is not whether pain has a voice or appearance: the question is whether those people who insist that it does not are interested in what pain has to say, and whose bodies are doing the talking.

Boyer exposes the exculpatory ableism behind characterizations of pain as indescribable rather than unpalatable or burdensome to apprehend. When pain is unspeakable, it remains invisible. The excessive appearance of pain invites a return to examining the historically specific—the cries and exclamations of the hysterics were certainly thought to be expressions of pain, though from what, exactly, was unclear—to say nothing of the rhetorical difficulty of expressing the severity of *chronic* pain. One can only howl, cry, scream, shriek, or whimper for so long.

Try, if you can, to imagine the worst pain you have ever functioned through. That is to say, not the kind of acute pain that requires immediate attention, that which would have you taken in an ambulance to the emergency room, but the worst pain you've endured through, say, a normal day of work. A migraine, perhaps. How much time could you endure this pain? A week? A month? A year? Assuming you might experience a wave of relief before the return of this pain, ask yourself how long you could go between waves of relief before you started to question carrying on. My literary project of writing about pain is figuring out how to write a perpetual scream—that is, how to survive my life. Do I want to know, as Audre Lorde wrote of her motivation for finishing *The Cancer Journals*, that "the pain [will] not be wasted"? Or do I fear that writing about illness will soon be impossible? Hélène Cixous said in a published interview, "But I think the only thing that could paralyze one's writing is a fettering, an arrest of the subject inside themselves. It can happen when one's life force is affected. And I tell myself very humbly that illness, true illness, the body's illness, which introduces a hostile and unfathomable stranger, can steal, strangle the live force of writing."

Daudet wrote that "pain is always new to the sufferer, but loses its originality for those around him." Another worthy literary project: to convey the perpetual *newness* of chronic pain.

The story of my illness doesn't exist. There are great spaces in which I can grasp at sign or origin, tracing the decline in ability about which I've already written, but I cannot say with certainty which parts of me have been or will be lost, what kind of knowing is available to me now. Investigations yield a book about being upset with the world, a book that is in itself upsetting, but so is what we ask an illness narrative to contain: the uncomfortable dance between the needy and the needed, the weight of a precarious life, the cries of ill embodiment, and the utter ordinariness of all these things that come for each of us eventually. An illness narrative must be sprung from a debt of vitality and love but must also offer vengeance against that which diminishes life.

What diagnosis *does* provide is discipline and practice. I watch myself constantly for signs of disease, signs that the body is in the midst of a flare and must be reined in with steroids or other immune-suppressing drugs.

Let's try again to tell the story: I am sick, possibly have always been sick, and now my sickness has a name. What should I do differently? For a newly diagnosed person with internet access, the suggested remedies are dizzying, endless, and offer little hope: Avoid caffeine. No alcohol or recreational drugs, ever. Expensive air purifiers I cannot afford might help with respiratory symptoms and rashes. I should use all organic, fragrance-free products in the home, and live in a home built before or after various years when toxin regulations changed. I should live far from cell phone towers. On top of my medications to manage pain and suppress immune response, I should take between ten and twenty supplements each day and chart how my body responds to each. I should adjust my expectations for myself, for my life: read only that which is short and succinct, comprehended through brain fog, spend nights in, surround myself only with those who understand the gravity of my illness, and take other, similar precautions. I should have access to resources, doctors, and services that would be possible only under fully automated luxury communism. Insurmountable.

I have come to recognize the sense of fatalism this engenders as emblematic of the particular tone of the life spent sick. Suddenly, you can't smile or laugh or find joy or hope in anything. To a healthy person, it might look like depression.

Contrary to popular belief, there are many great books about illness. My favorites are those that make a literary space out of illness, make material out of brain fog, show the fragmentary texture of thought-in-pain, thought subject to medications, plots punctuated by blood draws, the embarrassment of attempting to communicate through declining cognitive ability, the fundamental question of what to do with an unsaved life.

Following the success of his 1990 book, *To the Friend Who Did Not Save My Life*, and his rapid deterioration due to AIDS, Hervé Guibert stopped writing. Perhaps he no longer needed the money, or didn't think he could outdo its success, or simply couldn't lift his water glass. Guibert had been ambivalent about whether he wanted to know if he was seropositive for HIV: what was the point, he wondered, when such knowledge could drive someone like him to suicide? His book, a roman à clef of his experience being diagnosed with and losing friends to AIDS, was a scandalous release in France, largely because it revealed the death of "Muzil," a thinly veiled Michel Foucault, to have been caused by AIDS. Guibert writes an extended portrait of his friend and mentor's last days and wonders if it is a betrayal to do so. Foucault's writing on the medical gaze is illuminated by Guibert's portrayal of him: Muzil "told me he'd forgotten how completely the body loses all identity once it's delivered into medical hands, becoming just a package of helpless flesh, trundled around here and there, hardly even a number on a slip of paper."

Guibert chose not to hide his illness the way Foucault did. *To the Friend Who Did Not Save My Life* becomes the project of documenting the illness. Early on, Guibert writes that even once he sensed the structure of the book, he imagined multiple endings, and that "the whole truth is still hidden from me, and I tell myself that this book's raison d'être lies only along this borderline of uncertainty, so familiar to all sick people everywhere." Along the borderline of uncertainty, illness's plot is revealed: Illness progresses. Friends react. Quack doctors and naturopaths capitalize on the finitude of the vulnerable. Each blood draw brings with it information: depletion of T4 cells, a prescription for AZT—a kind of ending, because someone about to take the drug is "already dead, beyond hope of salvation." Rightfully, Guibert does not grasp at lessons or wisdoms to be passed on to the next generation of sufferers or to the healthy, but instead documents the illness, "sleek and dazzling in its hideousness, for though it was certainly an inexorable illness, it wasn't immediately catastrophic, it was an illness in stages, a very long flight of steps that led assuredly to death, but whose every step represented a unique apprenticeship. It was a disease that gave death time to live and its victims time to die, time to discover time, and in the end to discover life."

He also does not, as was the case with Muzil, seek out morbid silver linings: "Between fits of coughing," Muzil "was eager to report on his latest escapades in the baths of San Francisco. That day I remarked to him, 'Those places must be completely deserted now because of AIDS.' 'Don't be silly,' he replied, 'it's just the opposite: the baths have never been so popular, and now they're fantastic. This danger lurking everywhere has created new complicities, new tenderness, new solidarities. Before, no one ever said a word; now, we talk to one another. We all know exactly why we're there.'"

It's easy to see why, given such character sketches, Guibert felt closer to selling out his friends when he wrote about them versus when he photographed them. The novel charts his own exorbitant efforts to leverage his celebrity status to procure special treatment and be cured by an experimental vaccine, so no one is depicted especially charitably. More striking is the way in which solidarity among Muzil and his friends creates, to some degree, the ability to live.

The term *la belle indifférence*, used to describe a strange lack of concern about one's own illness, particularly in patients of hysteria or conversion disorders, gained popularity after Freud used it to describe 'Elisabeth von R' in *Studies in Hysteria*. It isn't clear how useful this categorization is as a diagnostic criterion, but it's largely considered to be part of the broader phenomenon of anosognosia, or "denial of illness." An example given to students studying for the psychiatric board is that of a man who suddenly goes blind after the death of his mother. No physical cause for his blindness can be found, and the man is completely unconcerned with his inability to see. This hints to his caretakers that he may be a conversion patient.

Is the lack of concern really so strange? Might it be a way of telling oneself one story so as to avoid another? The kind of frantic grasping-at-the-life-force that happens when pain sets in might look like carelessness, but I think of it as grieving in advance, as clinging to shards of the peak experiences of life that you might lose access to too young. It is why, even after receiving a diagnosis, I continue to live, whenever possible, as I like—in denial, perhaps, but also, occasionally, liberated. When I can do it, it's easy: the invisibility of my disease is on my side, after all, especially after a round of steroids, which give me an insatiable appetite and the edge of a healthier appearance through a few extra pounds. While I resist the idea of intoxicants being "for" anything, I couldn't agree more with William James that they offer clear benefits for those whose pain has no end in sight—when Alice was diagnosed with breast cancer, he urged her to "take all the morphia (or other forms of opium if that disagrees) you want, and don't be afraid of becoming an opium-drunkard. What was opium created for except times such as this?"

Sections of the book you're reading now were written on opiates, with amphetamines to push through the opiate haze, steroids to suppress flares, benzos to temper the steroid frenzy, and various other drugs causing nausea—for which marijuana (which I called "slacker Xanax" in my ballet days) is, unfortunately, the only effective antidote I have found. Various intoxicants and the relief they offer allow me to be okay—okay because I *want* to be okay, to be able to drink and eat and have a social life and forget pain once in a while, even at great delayed cost; or okay because I *have* to be to keep my job to keep my health care to treat my disease. In either case, I cannot handle as much as other people can. In both cases, I must appear well enough not to draw concerned attention to myself. Both are fake. Both are temporary. Only the former, in combination with the ideal substances, provides the mania of feeling okay. You can spend your whole life with a voracious appetite and then, when the tide of chronic illness comes in, no longer desire food or sex or art or even mind-numbing, frivolous distraction—and it doesn't matter too much. You just have to wait for the tide to ebb; for desire for something, anything, to return. I binge and purge health.

Guibert's final entry: "My book is closing in on me. I'm in deep shit. Just how deep do you want me to sink? . . . My muscles have melted away. At last my arms and legs are once again as slender as they were when I was a child."

When I can't get my thoughts down, I look at the photographs of Augustine. In one, she is mischievous, giving Charcot a sidelong glance, skeptical, and I wonder if she so obediently offered herself up for medical policing not only to create a beautiful final photograph or contribute knowledge about the nature of her illness, but also to experience the time spent posing, the moment of self-loss, respite, oblivion. Are the images a quickened path to the climaxes of her life? Does she have a clear image of herself outside Charcot's creation?

Augustine continues to come to me; I continue to transcribe her; we are united in having been rendered in a language that cannot account for us. It is too easy to speculate about her motivations. It is entirely possible that she found the life available to her before the Salpêtrière banal, that the possibilities of a life in the confines and language of the hospital were simply more exciting. The retreat of bodyminds from an unacceptable world, the scream of symptoms against chemicals and contagion—both create the conditions of refusal: I am constantly discovering new things I cannot or will not do.

Or maybe it was about the taking of the picture, the process and the ritual, the feeling that the act of being photographed was what she *was*, if who we are is how we fill the vastness of our days. Or, maybe—and this is the explanation I favor most—maybe she followed Charcot into that studio for each private rehearsal enthusiastically, her eyes locked on him the whole time, and when she slipped into the passionate poses for the camera, she was triumphant. She was getting precisely what she wanted, and if I watch her closely enough, I might, too. But, of course, the most likely explanation is an ancient, thoughtless instinct toward survival.

I prefer Augustine's photographs to accounts of her life and symptoms, written by doctors, labeling her poses and attacks. In the archive of her photos, her face is appropriated but also drawn down from clinical anonymity. Am I simply punctum hunting through her photos, limiting their significance to whatever they make me feel, whatever they present to me about myself? In graduate school, I wrote a contrived paper modeling such a hunt. In W. G. Sebald's *Austerlitz*, the title character recalls observing a woman he believes to be his mother, who was forced to appear in a Nazi propaganda film: "Around her neck, she is wearing a three-stringed and delicately draped necklace which scarcely stands out from her dark, high-necked dress, and there is, I think, a white flower in her hair . . . I gaze and gaze again at that face, which seems to me both strange and familiar, said Austerlitz, I run the tape back repeatedly." I wrote that I was waiting for something, a rupture in Austerlitz's examination of the film as a pure document, but all I was able to find is that he described the necklace incorrectly; in fact, it had only two strings, an occurrence that bears an uncanny similarity to Roland Barthes's error in *Camera Lucida*: Barthes misdescribes the necklace in a James Van Der Zee photo as a set of braided gold ribbons when it was actually a string of pearls—significant, given that the author identifies this necklace as his punctum in the photograph, the prick that ruptures his experience of concentrated observation. For Barthes, the punctum could not be willed; it is the accident that wounds. When the viewer approaches a photograph searching for such an accident, what is found is perhaps always destined to be of themself. Is it possible for me to surrender to Augustine's photos, premeditating nothing, wanting nothing, receiving her only as she presented herself? What of her has pricked me? What can the photos be to me; what can they do? I am tortured, looking for a punctum to devour. I want to create a vocabulary, make her into words, but can only continue to inscribe what I see in her images.

I can't provide a history of my illness, but I can provide a history of jobs I've done while sick and an account of what they cost me. Most of these employers preemptively sidestepped any legal obligation to accommodate the sick or disabled, by (illegally) hiring full-time workers as independent contractors. Most had no idea I had health problems—until I was forced to tell them, sometimes from a hospital bed. When one's illness cannot be made visible, one's entire life changes in secret. Having aged out of my first two careers of ballet and modeling, I found that the ways in which I *was* visible in my early twenties perhaps rendered my illness even less perceptible.

One summer in my early twenties, I edited for one of the last surviving fashion and culture print magazines on the West Coast. In my interview, the editor, who wore a gold cocaine spoon dangling from his neck, had recognized me from evenings spent at the Chateau Marmont, where he liked to hang out with the blondest, straightest boys and where I liked to people-watch and see if I couldn't acquire some mania of feeling okay. I expected to hate the magazine job. I did not expect it to carry the expectation of more-than-full-time work for less money than my graduate school stipend, or that everyone on staff would smoke indoors. *You should have seen it a few years ago,* my coworkers said over my coughing fits. *They used to make the interns take Adderall so they could work longer.* They warned me that when it came time to close an issue, I'd be expected to work overnight to have it ready for the printers on time. I knew the cigarette smoke was a likely trigger for my vasculitis, but I didn't see the point in complaining until I had another job lined up. The smoke gave me chronic throat infections. *There are no ethical jobs under capitalism,* I thought. I still had health care, but I had to work for it, and I sensed that the time I could spend living off truffle fries and cocktails that someone else paid for and selling the free designer clothing I had acquired was waning.

I spent a lot of time that summer on the rooftop of another nearby hotel, owned by a friend. I liked going there—you have to get really high above the city for Los Angeles to present as having any kind of order or plan. The women were proudly Eurotrashy, and the men dressed like rich older women, in nylon Prada suits with crystal brooches and silk smoking loafers. I liked the sweet relief of their platitudes, which, without cocaine or a comparable intoxicant, I would have found unbearable—about Moon Juice, Botox, twelve-step programs, and the character of the city, "Los Angeles." I wanted that levity. A small group who often found each other on the roof liked to ask me about writing and media. One night, when the pain crept back in hours after I'd popped a Tramadol, when I knew that anything stronger would slow me down, I found myself bending over the little mirrored tray in the rooftop bathroom to do the line of cocaine being offered to me by a stunning designer I'd met about five minutes before. She told me she liked my haircut, that it was the Jane Birkin cut she'd always wanted, but she couldn't pull it off because she has a cowlick where the fringe should be. I told her how I used to have her haircut—jaw-length and slicked back, like the famous photo of Isabella Rossellini taken while some guy lights her cigarette—which made us laugh. The designer wasn't going to do coke tonight herself, she said, but given that I liked it so much, she thought she might as well—it was hard to find cool girls to talk to, she said with a heavy sigh. Surely, I must have remembered this from my modeling days.

I did remember, so I nodded and laughed again. With each line, I could become more gregarious and benevolent, so I could keep having conversations like this one, despite the pain coursing through my body. Strictly speaking, I was not supposed to do coke at all—even more than any normal person isn't supposed to—because of the drug's inflammatory effect on the blood vessels, but cocaine reinstates the desire to do everything and know everything and be everywhere that is marred by pain and painkillers. I missed it. And I was good at it: I took steady, conservative amounts, experienced no comedown or blues, and slept soundly afterward. It would be a shame for an affinity like that to go to waste.

The designer and I swaggered out of the bathroom and toward the rooftop fireplace to rejoin our group. We sat down on the chaises longues under a big fur throw blanket and ordered another round of drinks. As someone rolled a joint, the rooftop started to spin. Not spin like I'd gotten too high or had had too much to drink, but spin like I was about to lose consciousness. Sounds blended together, ringing echoed off the inside of my skull, the lights of the neighborhood swirled together magnificently. *No matter*, I thought. *I've learned to accommodate this*. I eased myself back on my elbows and curled up into a relaxed fetal position that I hoped might be seen as playful. When I saw a look of concern spread over several people's faces, it occurred to me that I should tell them the name of my disease, in case I did faint—I'd had less-than-ideal experiences at urgent care centers whose doctors had never heard of it, much less knew how to interpret its inflammatory effects wreaking havoc on my body, whatever state it was in.

I'm probably just tired, I explained, careful to keep my tone calibrated to a dismissal, not a plea, *but it* might *be this other thing. I think I'll head home soon.*

I heard my voice float up into the air around me, which felt somehow laden with surfaces. There was something in the designer's eyes then, something hard to name. Finally, it came to me: pity. She felt sorry for me.

She said, *Oh, I didn't know you were ill—maybe we shouldn't have been doing those lines.*

Someone else asked if I'd tried Reiki. Other members of the group nodded, offering various wellness efforts that they believed to have healed them or others: gluten-free diets, cutting out all drugs but recreational ones, an energy healer on the coast, something called "setting intentions on the highest possibilities."

You mean positive thinking? I asked. *What I think about my disease doesn't seem to have much to do with it at all.*

To live and die in LA is to be surrounded by self-absorption sold as virtue. Why focus on the minutiae of my suffering, microcosms of worry, when I could do something to achieve temporary transcendence?

On my way home, my dizziness resolved—a close call—so I stopped for a Mai Tai at one of the many tiki bars that claimed to have created the drink. If you haven't spent much time in Hollywood—not East or West Hollywood, but Hollywood Hollywood—the thing is that the days of Eve Babitz are long gone, and it's quite grungy and meta-nostalgic: everything is decorated to make it seem like you are somewhere in the middle of the last century, but the only places that have been around that long can be rather bleak. I sucked down the slushy drink and took in the scene: tourists and the elderly who had been haunting those hot-pink vinyl seats for fifty years, illuminated together under neon lights and plastic toucans.

Later that summer, at lunch with friends, I did lose consciousness, hitting my head on the concrete ground. While I had long understood that my adolescent fainting spells had been caused by neuro-Behçet's, this time, I got my first abnormal MRI reading—it suggested that my fainting spell had brought with it brain damage. Was it that I'd spent the summer overworked in a hot oven of cigarette smoke? Was it the occasional partying I'd come to rely on for morale? When someone in the throes of chronic illness experiences flares as unavoidable, only ever delayed, the details can feel too superficial to have much bearing on the illness's overall trajectory. Nevertheless, I resolved to rein in the partying and quit the job at the magazine. A few years later, an assistant sued the CEO and editor in chief for sexual harassment. According to the suit, when the assistant confronted the offender about several events of harassment, the offender promised to separate professional and personal relationships and to stop doing cocaine with the interns.

While working as a staff writer at a progressive news site funded and published by an heiress, I called in sick one day from the hospital, in the midst of a horrible flare. *Take as much time off as you need*, the heiress told me. *Rest. Heal.* Rent was due the following week. I could not take any time off if I was going to continue to live under a roof or be able to pay the premiums on my subsidized freelancer's healthcare plan. Fighting to breathe, to lower my fever, to feel the steroids coursing through my veins so that I might remain conscious, I'd lost the luxury of righteous class anger. Nothing was unexpected anymore because I no longer had expectations; nothing was killing me because I was already dying. Several years later, the heiress folded the publication rather than grant the remaining staff's rather modest labor demands, like compensation for healthcare costs, paid vacation days, and new contracts to reflect California labor laws.

There are those who can afford rest and the healing that might come with it and those who must try perilously to steal them.

It is perplexing that health is so often thought of as ancillary to labor, class, and racial struggles, when it intersects so profoundly with each. As a crime reporter at a daily regional newspaper in college, I became acquainted with the linguistic similarities by which these struggles are obfuscated. I was taught to use passive phrases in my articles—"in an *officer-involved shooting* a man died at least partially due to his *pre-existing condition*"—which asserted a relief-laced logic: only *that* person will die because of the aberration of their individualized flaw. When someone has a preexisting condition, they are biologically irredeemable; their death cannot be entirely the fault of whoever or whatever killed them. It's the kind of language we analyze in the medical humanities courses I now teach: a recent newspaper article on the Covid-19 pandemic recently reframed *preexisting conditions* as "pulling deaths from the future": "Researchers will be studying if the COVID pandemic may be 'pulling deaths from the future,' hastening the deaths of people who were nearing death, though that will not be evident for several months." The creation of distinctions between the social value of a lost "normal" life versus the perhaps closer-to-death "sick" life paints the deaths of the most vulnerable people as preordained. Artist Beatrice Adler-Bolton writes that "the idea that any of the death and despair that vulnerable populations have seen throughout the duration of the pandemic is necessary has been manufactured through frameworks of austerity. This results in deadly political inaction that threatens the survival of vulnerable people and will impact their health outcomes not just during the pandemic but for decades to come."

In *Illness as Metaphor*, Sontag warns against using the former as the latter, to avoid not only linguistic slipperiness, but also the manner in which illness comes to stand for the culture's fear du jour. AIDS stood for a fear of sex and homosexuality, cancer for the perceived repression that was punitively associated with it. Xenophobia is now embedded in what some call pandemics—the *Spanish* flu, the *Chinese* virus. The English called syphilis the French disease, the French called it the Neapolitan disease, and the Neapolitans said it came from America, where colonizers had been infected by the "Indians." The headaches, fatigue, and cognitive dysfunction often present in autoimmune diseases and invisible illnesses are charged with interpretation: Derrida argued that the idea of democracy suffered from a fatal "autoimmunity," in that its requirements for freedom and equality canceled each other out. (This metaphor seems more closely aligned with the medical definition of HIV infection, in which the immune system destroys itself, than with that of autoimmune disease, in which the immune system targets the body's organs. In any event, the body/body politic contains within itself the possibility of its own undoing.)

Sontag wrote a little-known play on Alice James, *Alice in Bed*, in which she merges the character Alice James with Lewis Carroll's Alice. James, who, in addition to physical ailments, suffered deep depression beginning at a young age, unsuccessfully attempts to gain her father's consent to kill herself. ("But you're not trying to want something else," he says to her.) In the first scene, she argues with a nurse about whether she "can't" or "won't" get out of bed, where she spends her time immobilized but mentally abuzz. In an opium dream-like state, Alice is visited by women from nineteenth-century literature and by Myrtha, the queen of the Wilis in *Giselle*, who offers her counsel at a tea party. Myrtha offers to kill Alice's father, freeing her from the cage of his desire for her to live. "I always thought a man would crush me," Alice replies. "He would put a pillow over my face. I wanted a man's weight on my body. But then I couldn't move."

Was it the man crushing Alice James, or was it life in the trenches of mind-body medicine? Even more scientifically minded thinkers like William James believed that the laws of faith healing could be studied and harnessed—he called the "mind cures" of the New Thought movement "the religion of healthy-mindedness," and Charcot cited faith healings as evidence that the mind could extend its influence into the functions of physiology. The movement, which suggested that, through faith or the power of positive thinking, patients could alter the course of disease, was particularly popular with women eager to see their "intuitiveness" channeled toward improving their physical frailty. Alice found suggestions that she think more positively about her illness as exasperating as I do. She wrote to William in 1899 that she felt even more ill after a surprise visit from a woman who followed the teachings of the movement, who had insisted Alice's symptoms were due not to her physical state but to her mind. "When I asked her what attitude of the mind was that she assumed in her wrestle with fate," she wrote, "the poor lady cd. not make an articulate sound . . . she finally murmured 'to lose oneself in the Infinite,' wh. process seems to bring one rather successfully to the surface in the finite as the Curer 'says her power is the same as Christ's only less perfect.'"

It is peculiar that Alice's symptoms were interpreted with the excess of hysteria, when her attitude toward her illness is clear, unsentimental—she was *resigned* to the life of an invalid. Toward the end of her life, she looked back on her illness's trajectory: "As I lay prostrate after the storm with my mind luminous and active and susceptible of the clearest, strongest impressions, I saw so distinctly that it was a fight simply between my body and my will, a battle in which the former was to be triumphant to the end." Suggestions that a patient who has accepted this corporeal reality try to heal through the power of their mind strike me as particularly punitive. The doctor who gently suggested I recalibrate my expectations, that I might never again feel "close to one hundred percent," did more for my self-understanding than any civilian attitude or dietary proposition.

Chronic illness brings with it a terrible amount of anxiety: *I am in pain; there will likely be more pain; I might always feel this pain.* Yet, paying obsessive attention to the pain of symptoms is stressful; and stress makes the patient more susceptible to further flares of illness. Disease both reacts to stress and creates it. Genuinely accepting illness, without hope of futurity, is hard-won. It was not in her attitude but in her journal that Alice found a means of controlling the narrative of her illness: "I shall at least have it all my own way and it may bring relief as an outlet to that geyser of emotions, sensations, speculations and reflections, which ferments perpetually within my poor carcass for its sins."

Todd Haynes's 1995 film *Safe*, set in 1987, deep in the trenches of the Reagan years, opens with sweeping views of the San Fernando Valley from inside a black Mercedes: manicured lawns and mid-century architecture, a landscape that is pristine yet ominous enough to warrant that it might become a threat to our middle-aged, incredibly passive housewife protagonist, Carol (played by Julianne Moore). Carol speaks in a high-pitched, breathy Valley accent, struggles with small talk, and does not appear to have meaningful bonds with those around her. She seldom completes a sentence. (Could

saying nothing be the same as saying no?) Carol's conversations are strained; each ellipsis of her silence is loaded; yet it
is through her symptoms that her character is most revealed.
She believes she has contracted an environmental illness
because she experiences physical symptoms when she is
around certain everyday chemicals—has difficulty breathing,
gets a nosebleed while at the hair salon. Her emptied-signi-
fier trajectory is familiar: the men around her believe she is a
hysteric; the family doctor insists nothing is wrong with her or
believes her suffering to be psychosomatic. Eventually, Carol
has a complete collapse at a store that has been fumigated
with pesticides. She now believes she can no longer continue her current life and moves to Wrenwood, a New Age
alternative treatment community in the desert, led by a charismatic leader named Peter, a "chemically sensitive person with
AIDS." At Wrenwood, Carol's illness is believed and affirmed,
though the familiar New Age story about sickness being the
result of one's thoughts and feelings still reigns: at one point,
Peter tells his charges that "the only person who can make you
sick is you," nearly quoting New Age writer Louise Hay's *The
AIDS Book: Creating a Positive Approach*. It makes sense that
Hay, whose writing career began with the small pamphlet *Heal
Your Body* (a list of different bodily ailments and their "probable" corresponding metaphysical causes), was an inspiration
for Haynes's alluring leader, who urges people to take responsibility for how sick they are.

We never find out what is wrong with Carol. Some critics
have taken issue with Haynes's ambiguity, but this strikes me
as the film's greatest strength: whatever Carol's illness is, it does

not lend itself to a tidy narrative in the way that "real" physical or psychosomatic disease might. Her condition could improve, only for her to succumb to another immobilizing flare. If her illness is granted a name, it could only serve as a restatement of the problem. She will continue to be interpreted—by doctors, by her fellow Wrenwood inhabitants, and by herself—through the prismatic lens of biology and biography. Carol struggles with Wrenwood's characteristic language and is apologetic that she is "still learning, you know, the words." Asked to give a speech at a communal meal, she stutters, "I really hated myself before I came here . . . I'm trying to see myself, hopefully, more as I am, more, um, more positive, like seeing the pluses?" I can't imagine what those might be. For the viewer, Carol's failure to internalize Wrenwood's teachings looks like a triumph of sorts, and even in the film's final scene, as she struggles to say "I love you" to her reflection in a mirror, the red rash across her fore-head speaks louder than her trembling voice.

When one simply cannot accept the impossible terms of forever illness, the idea that something, anything, can be done might be of comfort, no matter how shrouded in utter bullshit it may be. Louise Hay's New Age doctrine isn't far off from the positive thinking, self-help, and salvation-as-commodity flouted by the modern wellness industry—while some patients understand that positive thinking won't cure illness, most people believe some version of my doctor's assertion that "the mind and body interact in mysterious ways" and that these "ways" are receptive to some manipulation brought about by our choices or actions. Health-as-capital holds the individual consumer accountable for whatever might go wrong with their body: if they tried the right product, followed the right diet, *took responsibility for their illness*, they wouldn't be so sick. Yet, it isn't difficult to see why a sick person, someone on the margins, with few alternatives, might cling to the possibility of healing. Conspiracy thrives when reality becomes unbearable. It is the experience of seeking treatment for her illness that pushes Carol toward an examined life, even when—or, per-haps, because—the purported recovery requires a retreat from the stakes and conditions of the world.

When suffering is met with insufficient language, people sometimes, especially in Los Angeles, come together to create a new one. At a party, a friend told me I *had* to visit her healer, a man on the coast whose practice is advertised entirely by word-of-mouth. He works with celebrities, coaches, athletes, and was himself a former Olympic swimmer. When my friend could not get pregnant, she started seeing him to "realign" her "whole situation." She believes it worked, and calls this man "the real father" of her child. The "suggested donation" for a session with this healer was about equivalent to my monthly rent at the time. I, a sensible person with a veritable, medically specific illness, did not want to see this healer, but soon after the party, the healer's wife, who handles his appointments, called to schedule a session that I had been gifted.

It's fine, I told myself—*it's normal, often quite reasonable, to be deeply distrustful of biomedicine, especially in LA.* I had recently interviewed a wellness guru who believed that clean eating had cured her lupus and inspired her "chemical-free" skincare line. My friends go on meditation retreats; raise their children on gluten-free diets; breastfeed their verbal toddlers; do Ayurvedic cleanses, past-life regression, bee sting therapy, raw food diets. My grandmother practices Reiki and used to wave her arms above me as I lay in bed, sending the badness out of my body. This wasn't even the first time in recent memory I'd been given a quack treatment as a gift: I'd recently completed a cryogenic freezing session "where the Lakers do it"—"it" ostensibly being "reducing inflammation and diseased tissue through locking yourself in a freezer for a controlled amount of time." Cryotherapy's effectiveness has not been demonstrated in controlled studies, and my session considerably exacerbated my Raynaud's symptoms, because . . . duh. Countless friends have recommended Transcendental Meditation or body scanning, which aims to release unrealized tension by focusing on individual body parts, moving gradually from the feet to head. I find this doesn't relieve tension so much as it makes me hyperaware of all the locations of pain and their corresponding tensions that I will be unable to correct. I usually take a painkiller after an attempt at "body scanning," and the pains of each different body part start to soften around the edges and bleed together. I sometimes say that opiate painkillers don't "kill" pain so much as make everything so foggy you don't notice your pain in the same way, taking any lucidity of thought, feeling, or sound with them. This seems the most I should hope for.

Debates about biomedical versus alternative treatments for autoimmune conditions—like those concerning vaccinations—purport to be about science, but they might as well be about power. We think of a charlatan as someone who preys upon the weak and desperate, but so many people are suffering under a system that will not offer them relief that entire cottage industries create themselves to offer it. People in pain can be forced to make decisions out of desperation, and when the only options offered in the health-as-capital economy are terrible, it can be difficult to do an effective comparative analysis as a health "consumer." Alternative healing modalities often profess that the material and immaterial parts of a person are enmeshed and that thoughts and feelings affect the body on a physical level. While this is frustrating, it isn't inherently any more absurd than cognitive behavioral therapy's belief that our thoughts, and not external material circumstances, cause our feelings and behaviors. This is what I told myself, repeatedly, before I went to see the healer. What did I have to lose? (The health consumer *always* has something to lose.)

I was running late. It was a hot day, and the freeway was sprinkled with convertibles with their tops down. When I finally approached the manicured, unironically palm-lined lawns of the neighborhood, my unease had evolved into pure, unadulterated dread. As instructed, I followed the path to a house where the man whom I presumed to be the healer—I'll call him John—was sitting on one of the sofas. The other sofa, apparently, was for me. I apologized profusely for my lateness as I shook his hand—a gesture he seemed to find puzzling—and noticed that he had been sitting there entirely unoccupied, perhaps basking in his own undiluted mindfulness. *Stop being such an asshole. You came into this with an "open mind."* There were no TV or computer screens in the room, but there was some cheesy pop music playing lightly in the background. I was not sure where it was coming from.

The way John's eyes shifted up and down my person reminded

me not so much of ogling by sleazy men but, rather, the unsettling, quick assessment of certain newly-introduced women.

That's a short dress, he said to me, eyes still flicking. *It tells me something about the kind of attention you're seeking.*

(This is when I should have walked out.)

I told him it was a gift from the designer—dry-clean only—and that the only thing it should indicate to him was that I'd been too overworked and sick to do laundry.

Good thing that what I do is growth and healing, he continued. *Whatever has messed you up Out There, In Here, we'll take care of it.*

Growing up, I always admired kids who, when forced into therapy, refused to speak, recognizing the betrayal that language would be to themselves and whatever landed them there in the first place. That I-would-prefer-not-to refusal. I, on the other hand, have done a lot of therapy, and as my continual submission to the medical gaze suggests, I err on the side of "compliant." So when John asked, *Okay, what's the problem?* the words tumbled out of my mouth with the ease of an elevator pitch that has been rehearsed countless times:

I have an autoimmune disease. My illness is the most significant strain on my friendships and relationships. I indulge vices and people who allow me to forget that I am sick and will become sicker. I am then sometimes unable to return their expectations of intimacy—I've led them on, the person they like spending time with is not someone I am always able to be. I do not let lovers near my illness; I am only a lover when I am well enough. We only speak of illness in order to participate in a practical exchange of information—sorry, under the weather tonight, I can't make it after all. I find it more gracious than putting someone in the position of having to decide if being around my sickest self would be too much, too difficult for them: to my arms-length friends, I am kept in an imaginary state of health. I prefer to think of myself this way, too. I do not feel equipped to make medical decisions, given that I often cannot find any distinctions between the medical interventions that have saved my life and those that have caused me irreparable harm. Writing is the first thing that has made my life feel meaningful since ballet, and I am haunted by the ghost of my capable body, by my thinning hair and ruddy complexion, which worsens with each round of steroids. Last but not least, it disgusts me even to speak of these things, but they define the very essence of my life.

John had barely blinked since I began speaking. *Your disease,* he said, in a tone that suggested he did not believe what I had was a disease at all, *it's inflammatory in nature, correct?*

I confirmed that it was.

Inflammation, he said, *is* heat. *Sexual energy creates* heat. *You must have had sex very young. When a young woman ignites that fire too soon, it courses through her for the rest of her life. I bet that explains why these "illnesses" occur so much more frequently in women!* He kept his hands folded as he spoke, then he raised one to stroke his chin, awaiting my response.

Stunned but not surprised, I explained about the gene, the biomarker, the thing that presents my illness as "legitimate" to both doctors and quacks like John, feeling a twinge of guilt for perpetuating the biomarker-as-legitimacy paradigm. I offered up some potentially relevant information without heeding his evidentiary demand of confession: *I was an intense child. I approached the world with an intellectual fury, felt very deeply, liked extremely demanding physical activities. Doctors have confirmed that dance had a negative impact on my arthritic state.*

It's nothing to be ashamed of, John assured me, as though one could tell someone they were made sick by sex they had as a child without an ethical underscore. *You were full*—he was gesticulating now—*of young, vital energy, the kind only young women have. He was a vampire, drawing that energy, and now you're paying the price for it, with this heat, coursing through your body.*

I tried not to sigh, but I did, followed by a joke about how he seemed not to have learned too much from the Satanic panic and the danger of suggesting false memories, huh?

He stared at me blankly.

I was uncomfortable, and so offered one final acquiescence: *I understand what you mean, in a sense. My body does seem haunted by something.* (People who buy into this sort of thing tend to assume that there must be a past dark enough to have created such a shit show.)

Your friend who sent you here, he began again, *has suggested that you still live somewhat promiscuously.* Another sigh. *I'm piecing together a pattern of promiscuous behavior,* he said. *You're still affected by the heat.*

Sure, I replied, *I can very much see that is what you are piecing together.*

Despite John's rehearsed, authoritative calm, I assumed he was as uncomfortable as I was—we were essentially completely uninterested in speaking to each other; we found each other discursively wayward; there was no way we could have a conversation that sounded like anything but a demolition site. We both smiled stiffly.

He turned the cheesy pop music back on and guided me through some odd breathing exercises. It occurred to me that this was the first time I had discussed my illness, with anyone but a doctor, without speaking of Augustine. As I prepared to leave, he told me things would be different from now on, that I could expect not to be as sick.

John keeps, or tries to keep, a low profile. He has no website, no social media profiles. When I looked him up, the first result was a warning on a sketchy website that he was "a fraud and dangerous to your health." Apparently, he had been coaching a professional surfer in breathing exercises that bordered on self-asphyxiation. Minutes before the surfer entered the water in Topanga for a night surf, he had been texting with John's wife and doting secretary. He was later found facedown in the water, dead. The autopsy revealed that three major arteries to his heart were blocked. In the comments section of the article, former clients of John's shared their stories: One wrote that John "almost killed me and sexually assaulted me." Another said he had assaulted them as well. Still another said that in their single session with John, he "asked me coldly about my sexual history, including an inquiry about abortions (never had one) . . . I did weird breathing exercises that had me almost hyperventilating . . . [He] was way off. I found the experience violating and awful." Yet another client said John "almost killed me as well. I had to get a CT scan from almost breaking my skull open from these questionable practices. He also would touch me sexually when I was passed out or was fading out." Another: "He almost ruined my life."

What "healers" like John believe—that "the mind and body

interact in mysterious ways," that we repress trauma and it causes turmoil in the body—is, to some extent, accepted by both modern medicine and psychiatry. When New Age belief combines with dangerous methods, and the two don't appear to be altogether distinct from conventional "wisdom," what is to stop desperate, suffering people failed by the medical system from being subject to the control and domination of men like John? What about those who do not have access to medical insurance or disability, or whose illness has not yet been categorized and named? For patients who have found the bureaucratic, impersonal medical system unable to account for or alleviate their suffering, the focused attention of a pseudoscientific healer might be understandably enticing.

In *A Journal of the Plague Year*, technically a work of fiction, Defoe writes about Londoners' anticipation of the plague through a rise in astrology, fortune-telling, and pious prayer, disseminated through pamphlets and almanacs. While my diagnosis legitimizes my disease in the eyes of doctors and allows me access to treatment, much of what I am advised to endure as part of the course of treatment seems in denial of the societal conditions that enforce the illness. A person who experiences symptoms possibly tangled up in such a psychic conflict could pursue psychoanalysis—my reading of Freud on hysteria echoes that of many contemporary psychoanalysts: the hysteric's condition should not be interpreted as a divergence from a healthy norm but, rather, as protest against the existence of the norm itself—but psychoanalysis is seldom covered by medical insurance and is even less accessible to the average person than medical care.

If anything, my (albeit, often failed) attempts to have grace for friends who find solace in New Age thinking came from a realization: it took me years outside the ballet world to realize that when people made jokes about crazy aging ballerinas, they were talking about me, as I had been. Nothing looks quite so crazy from the inside.

A quick perusal of my syllabus for an undergraduate course in the medical humanities suggests myriad additional reasons people in underserved and marginalized groups hold warranted mistrust toward the medical establishment: the horrifying experiments conducted on enslaved Black people, attempts to justify slavery through "proven" racial difference; the Tuskegee syphilis experiments; the Puerto Rico contraceptive pill trials; forced sterilization of Native women; the spirometer; et cetera. My course closely examines the case of Henrietta Lacks, a Black woman who, despite not having given informed consent, provided the first immortalized human cell line while being treated for cervical cancer at Johns Hopkins in 1951. Lacks's family had heard stories about Black people being abducted by doctors after nightfall—stories of "night doctors" had circulated in their community since the 1800s, some of them told by enslavers to scare enslaved people into submission and others thought to have come from actual abductions for medical experiments. When the medical establishment has a long history of violence, it is no wonder patient-consumers lose their trust in it.

Recently, a friend told me she refused the Covid-19 vaccine because she believes Western medicine to be evil, inept, dehumanizing, driven by capital and not life, and in the pockets of Big Pharma. I could not disagree with her reasoning, only with her conclusion that the risks of the vaccine outweighed the benefits. Because so much of autoimmunity is speculated to be viral-onset, I suspected that young, generally healthy people who did not consider themselves at enormous risk would develop the long Covid symptoms that so closely resemble autoimmune disease: breathing problems, abdominal pain and digestive difficulty, fatigue, and general pain. Even when a large number of people experience the same collection of chronic symptoms, it's difficult not to be cynical about what it will take for them to be believed and treated. When my unvaccinated friend got Covid, I held my breath as she treated it only with herbs from an acupuncturist leading an herbal Covid treatment clinical trial at a new integrative medicine center granted a veneer of legitimacy through affiliation with the university system at which I teach. Public health measures are enacted through us, through our bodies, as they must be, but there are many directions in which one might point a finger of blame before settling on a population forced to be health consumers. The health consumer faces the very means of their staying alive being withheld for the benefit of capital and must then wade through the trenches of false dualisms—artificial/natural, self/outsider, public/private, left/right—while being expected, somehow, to exit with medical literacy.

I decided to make a pilgrimage to Augustine, to examine for myself the tangible places in which my uncertainty had long dwelled. But I had no money. I arranged an editing job with a magazine editor friend and stayed in my favorite hotel room in Paris: entirely black lacquer—the walls, the bathtub, everything—the ideal surface to render any powdered substances placed upon it as visible as possible. Even the ceiling was mirrored. The lacquer was a useful feature, as pills couldn't hit me quick enough to get me through a long day at the office, let alone the work that had actually brought me to Paris: finding Augustine, tracing her steps.

While it was the clinical images taken of Augustine that were most etched in my mind, Eugène Atget's famous 1909 photographs of the Salpêtrière courtyard are striking, and strikingly devoid of the hysterics, libertines, alcoholics, depressives, the poor, and otherwise undesirables who were dumped there after Louis XIV designated the structure, previously a gunpowder factory, as an asylum. Atget took his photographs, which required long exposure times, at dawn, when patients were asleep. "It is no accident that Atget's photographs have been likened to those of a crime scene," wrote Walter Benjamin. "Every passerby a culprit." Wandering the courtyard of the Salpêtrière after a long day of editing fashion credits and making cuts from interviews was anticlimactic in the opposite sense: far from hallowed ground, the site of Charcot's spectacular displays of hypnotized women of the *leçons du mardi matin* is still a functioning hospital complex, where a young woman on a Sebaldian quest for *something* cannot help but feel rather underfoot. Starting at Place Camatte Zaydoff and passing through the rue des Archers, I approached the housing structures that served as battalions and, soon, the place I was looking for, the Quartier des Folles: three long, narrow, one-story structures that had once housed six hundred hysterics in tiny, isolated cells, each with a respective pole in front of it, to which the hysterics, after an elaborate hygiene regimen, were chained for a daily allotment of fresh air.

These unlucky hysterics, who preceded Augustine and held no hope of her level of success in the hospital's culture, were freed, in a manner of speaking, by Dr. Philippe Pinel. The truth is less simple. Pinel sometimes expressed uncertainty that the mad patients were truly ill because of their ability to endure physical adversity as compared to the healthy, and he frequently reduced them to animality. In *Madness and Civilization*, Foucault wrote that Pinel marked a shift from physical to mental control and oppression, "by practicing a social segregation that would guarantee bourgeois morality a universality of fact and permit it to be imposed as a law upon all forms of insanity." By bringing physicians into the asylum, the medical enterprise became a moral project.

Charcot produced his hysteria photographs under the influence of a painting created twenty years before his birth, in

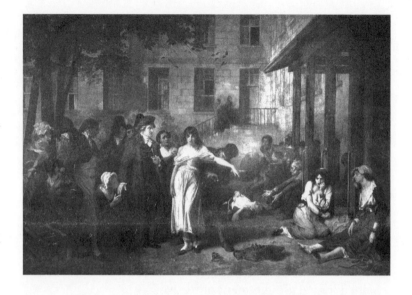

1805: Tony Robert-Fleury's *Pinel Liberating the Madwoman of the Salpêtrière*, depicting Doctor Pinel freeing a madwoman from her condition of solitary confinement. The woman being freed from her shackles seems hardly aware that this is the case: She stares off, looking in the general direction of the painter. She emotes little. She does not appear to be in great suffering, and this does not seem to be because she is being freed. She is nothing like the posed, well-lit women in the photographs of the hysterics. There is no pose of passion here, no ecstasy. Her hair and cream muslin dress are not arranged with any particular care. There are no giggle fits, no spasms. But directly below her left arm, which is being lifted by her liberator, we see a grotesque woman pulling her blouse open to expose one breast, her head thrown back. She is clamoring, crying, convulsing. She has already been freed of her chains, and those still enchained reach toward her, desperately. She has not been freed of her hysteria. She is so lost in the spectacle she has created that every onlooker appears to be a director. I think this is the woman-from-hell after whom Charcot modeled his own women when he took over, in his words, "the grand asylum of human misery," "the living museum of pathology" of the Salpêtrière.

A delivery truck pulled up behind the Quartier des Folles. A passing woman in a lab coat asked me without looking up from her cell phone, *Puis-je vous aider?*

I was embarrassed to be there, as if I were doing something wrong. The woman had a gap between her two front teeth that could be seen when she smiled—which she did when I was unable to answer her. *Bibliothèque Charcot?*

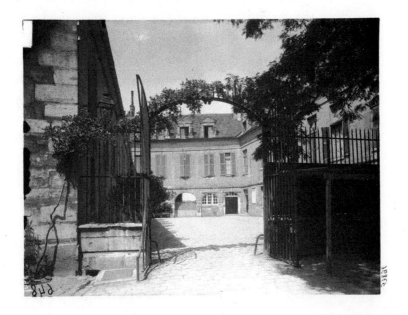

Her smile turned into an *ah* of recognition as she gave me directions. Sick young women, to whom the hysterics' stories might be somehow personal, sentimental, must go there often.

The amphitheater where Charcot's lessons were given no longer survives, but his library was donated to the hospital after his death. The books sit awkwardly in a tiny museum within a mid-century structure, where I felt a bit more at ease, alone, among the grass-and-resin scent of the old books—the lignin of old wood-based papers that is so closely related to vanillin. I didn't know what to ask for. Where might I find a mark, a sense, anything, of Augustine's living, breathing body? The Salpêtrière has been used unceasingly as a hospital; the ghosts haven't ever rested.

I felt too fragmented to speak French anymore. I lacked the perspective to decide which way to go. When I walked away from the hospital, not toward anything in particular, it appeared that its landscape was moving, too.

That night, I didn't want to stay in the hotel room alone, with all the stupid high-flash monochrome party photos of Dash Snow and Chloë Sevigny. I went downstairs to read Romanian philosopher Emil Cioran at the bar, with all the divorcées. I liked their clouds of ridiculous tuberose perfume and heavy Anna Karina kohl. The men hadn't bothered to dress with as much care, or maybe they had. What I was really doing was waiting for a man to come ask if I minded company and to invite me out for the night, which they always did—I liked this about Paris, the ease of the gendered expectations, not having to try. The serenity of drinking toward an approximation of a desire to spend an evening together.

Soon enough, a man with a drink in both hands introduced himself, said he couldn't help but notice that my Negroni was running low, and offered me one from his haul. When he asked what I did—even in Paris, one can't seem to escape the question—I told him I was a dental hygienist. It is the only response I have found that does not invite any follow-up questions; it is the kind of lie I tell all the time. He and I decided to leave the hotel bar to have dinner at a place he knew. As I reached for my wallet—my first mistake—he winced. Then I excused myself to go to the washroom to "powder my nose," an absurd, antiquated thing to say—my second mistake—where I instead crushed up a painkiller from my little pillbox so I would be able to endure the walk and the flavors of dinner.

In Saint-Germain-en-Laye, the *hôtels particuliers* have housed the same aristocratic families for generations. I decided against making a joke about class struggle. *They're too pristine*, I said, and explained that, having grown up in Southern California, I always suspected that such picturesque scenes might actually be soundstages. He laughed. When I asked for a cab back to the hotel after dinner, he placed his hand on my shoulder, heavily, to let me know he believed I was making a mistake. My third mistake.

Is it my age? he asked, dejected. He must have been about seventy. Many former ballerinas and former models I knew back in LA made a living dating men like him.

No, no, I assured him. *I'm just very focused on my novel. These long days working don't leave me much time to work on it.* I closed my eyes when I said the second part, as if, like a prayer, it might feel truer.

My novel! The line has stuck with me since. I use it often. While its authenticity as a romantic rejection might be questioned, it's more serviceable, more friendly than the actuality—I don't want anyone near how sick I am. Even now, after my illness has long had a name and, thus, has been called into medically-believed existence, when I speak of it, or hear someone speak in response, I never tell the whole story. On the rare occasions that I've tried, I've shuffled my feet, fidgeted with my watch, blushed, as though shame were attached to using words. Is it possible to be in pain without transmitting it to others? My sickness has given me the kind of ego that allows me to make someone feel unwanted and then to resent them for walking away.

In André Breton's 1928 surrealist novel *Nadja*, a man recounts ten days of obsession with the titular character, whom he meets on the street. He is fascinated with her through her vision of the world, which unfolds through discussion of surrealist artists like himself. Later in the book, Nadja is understood to be one of Pinel's mad patients. After she reveals details about her personal life, the man now fears she will disappoint him with her inability to live up to the fantasy he has built around her. Her symptoms have become so extreme that he must abandon her to forced institutionalization. The narrator then realizes his preference for ruminating on a memory of Nadja in which he can encounter her as a ghost—and better practice the theory of surrealism predicated upon the dreamlike nature of the experience of reality.

Léona Delcourt, the real woman on whom the character of Nadja was based, remained in psychiatric wards until her death in 1941. Breton's *Second Manifesto of Surrealism* opens with critical reactions to *Nadja* by psychiatrists. One of them, Gaëtan de Clérambault, developed a theory of mental automatism in psychotic delirium that led to additional scientific experiments in the physiology of stimulus-response.

Breton, who thought of hysteria as pure psychic automa-tism, said the condition was "characterized by the subversion of the relationships established between the subject and the moral world . . . It can, from every point of view, be considered as a supreme means of expression."

The final sentence of *Nadja*: "Beauty will be convulsive or not be at all." Augustine's violent, spastic beauty was an object of fascination for other surrealists as well, who saw hysteria as a state of idealized poetic expression. Her passionate poses were featured on the cover of the eleventh *La Révolution surréaliste*, a special "Research into Sexuality" issue. Breton called hysteria "the greatest poetic discovery of the late nineteenth century." The surrealists played automatic writing games, exercises in which they wrote "as if" they had conditions like hysteria, attempting to make the unconscious legible to themselves.

They used her for their ends. I am no different, reducing her life to these captured photography sessions. Does any of us know what we want from Augustine—to free her, diagnose her, consume her? To measure her against our own phys-ical deterioration, as I do? In any event, she rejected it all. During the last several months she spent at the hospital, she refused to allow Charcot to hypnotize her, refused to indulge the implicit idea that her submission to the medical gaze was part of a progressive and humane pursuit of knowledge. At this time, there is about her a sudden dimming in the photographs, a bereavement of sorts. She no longer appears a cheerful med-ical celebrity.

In her memoir written after the death of her husband, *The Year of Magical Thinking*, Joan Didion quotes Emily Post's 1922 book of etiquette, lauding the "unfailing specificity" of its practical advice for the needs of the mourner: "It is also well to prepare a little hot tea or broth, and it should be brought them upon their return without their being asked if they would care for it. Those who are in great distress want no food, but if it is handed to them, they will mechanically take it, and something warm to start digestion and stimulate impaired circulation is what they most need."

Rereading Didion's book, I found myself longing for something I had not realized I wanted: some kind of shared, specific, practical language for recognizing the needs of the ill; to be handed proverbial tea or broth without having to identify the desire for myself when I am enveloped in fire or fog; an invisible rupture of the healthy, neat public self I present to the world; an acknowledgment of the disparity. Without wading into diagnostics, it is easy to understand why the hysterics were inclined to use a visual language devoid of ambiguity about how to receive them. It's something I discussed with the late artist Carolee Schneemann: the elaborateness of Victorian mourning practices, colors and garments changed to

146 ~ Emily Wells

indicate to others who the deceased was to the mourner, the time since the death had elapsed. These traditions were rigid, and expensive, but there is a fundamental graciousness in visually signaling the specificity of one's distress to outsiders. Carolee, ever generous, spoke with me at length about writing this book. "Women's history has a special psychodynamic of burying all the social structures that really made women hysterical," she said. I think Freud would have agreed.

I can't get Augustine out of my head, I told my mother. It was a convenient, imprecise line.

So, what's the book about? she asked, to be polite.

My mind went blank; the fog set in, as though I were entirely unfamiliar with my object of obsession, naïve to her obvious significance and vibrancy. *It's the story of a woman who lacks the language to describe her physical experience,* I told her.

Yes?

The story of how she could not untangle her sick physical symptoms from her despair, from her memories, which constantly creep back in, haunt her.

Ah.

And she participated in a hospital culture of performance and spectacle in order to gain some small amount of power. It's all she can do, really: being this perfect, sick thing is essentially her job, which she's rather good at—following this charismatic doctor Charcot. She wants to get better, but she never does. We will never know the source of what condemns Augustine to these performances, to this life. The silence between us thickens. I wait for her to point out that I am really just trying to write about myself, but she doesn't.

The personal keeps seeping into the critical, refuses to be contained.

Augustine Gleizes is like all women of your generation, an older friend observed. *Splintered, fragmented.* On the one hand, she has quite tangibly improved her situation: she's managed to seduce the giant Charcot, seduces him through being the perfect case, making the perfect spectacle of her pain. She ensnares Charcot, keeps him, builds a life for herself at the Salpêtrière that is better, more exhilarating, more applauded than any life she could have had outside the hospital. On the other hand, she is the one who suffers from it all; she can no longer tell if her attacks are imitations of states of being, a glimpse of the true state of her body and mind, or something extracted, dragged out by Charcot.

My own life is made of fragments, and that's how it is with Augustine.

I returned only a few months later to Paris, to the Salpêtrière, to the lacquered hotel room, not as an "I" but as a "we," the other party constituting the "we" being a neuroscientist nervously practicing a talk about working memory to be given at an interview for a position across the country from where he lived—where I lived. He read a draft of a piece I was writing about Augustine and pointed out my tendency to slip into the passive voice when writing about myself. Berserk with vulnerability, I explained that this was reflective of how I experienced my illness as a force that directed both what I did and what happened to me, akin to the id. To write about my illness in the first-person active voice often feels only conditionally appropriate, expresses only one component of the situation in which I am also lived by illness.

As I climbed out of our room's bathtub one morning, a slab of marble broke and fell onto my foot. I did not need to explain the inflammatory aspects of my disease to my companion, as I had an injury to demonstrate them in real time. I felt that the episode might serve as an appropriate description about the way I lived—things fell apart around me, and from within me, and I tried with great force to achieve liminal states such that I might be able to push through them, often worsening the impact. The icy streets helped control the swelling as we walked—I hobbled—around the city, frenetic with excitement, speaking of, among many things, physiological markers and their role in the production of concepts, and Céline's medical dissertation: a novel about Ignaz Semmelweis, the Hungarian physician now thought of as the father of antisepsis, who was ostracized after suggesting that if physicians in Vienna's obstetrical clinics washed and disinfected their hands, their alarming fatality rates would decrease: "Semmelweis dashed himself against obstacles which, there is little doubt, most of the rest of us would have overcome by the exercise of simple prudence, and elementary politeness . . . In human terms, he lacked tact." The doctors found his suggestion insulting and mocked him. Semmelweis suffered a nervous breakdown and was committed to an asylum by his colleagues, where he died. Pasteur confirmed his germ theory years later.

I said, in jest, that the account reminded me of how Freud had written of *Nachträglichkeit*—or "afterwardsness," the idea that memory is in a sense "reprinted" in accordance with later experience—a century before scientists meaningfully studied memory reconsolidation; how, when scientists and clinicians spoke of Freud, it so often seemed as though they were describing an esoteric mystic who believed psyches to be detached from the physical processes of the body, instead of a materialist committed to the explanatory power of poetic gesture, as I had come to think of him. We have never stopped trying to describe these things to each other. Whenever an incision is made into the eternal entanglement of history and pathology, lives flood out and follow us like ghosts.

To think of the hysterics' madness as cries from the heart, an expression of some soulful artistry of women kept emotionally captive by their time and context, feels too easy, too literal. There is such strategy in the articulation of suffering of some women in pain that it can be difficult not to approach their words and images as art objects, but isn't an articulate strategy always demanded of a woman whose symptoms are not medically legible? What is she supposed to do but try to communicate the nature of her illness? Whether her culture understands her vocabulary has very little to do with it.

A dangerous dichotomy remains, then: What of Charcot, unable to help himself from documenting Augustine's beautifully expressed symptoms, her luxurious pain? Do I excuse myself from this atrocious paradox—am I not considering her actions as some sort of performance, accusing her of fabrication? The closest thing to a consensus on the images, from art historian Georges Didi-Huberman: "A reciprocity of charm was instituted between physicians, with their insatiable desire for images of Hysteria, and hysterics, who willingly participated and actually raised the stakes through their increasingly theatricalized bodies. In this way, hysteria in the clinic became the spectacle, the invention of hysteria. Indeed, hysteria was covertly identified with something like art, close to theater or painting." Huberman adds that he is "nearly compelled" to consider the Salpêtrière's hysteria spectacle as "a chapter in the history of art."

Hegel's chiasmus, the turning point, the catharsis, was incorporated by Pinel into the psychology of madness. The chiasmus says that madness is not a true loss of all reason, according to Hegel, but "a simple contradiction within reason," which, with human treatment, can be redirected, "just as physical disease is not an abstract, i.e., mere and total, loss of health (if it were that, it would be death), but a contradiction in it." But what is the chiasmus of Pinel's freed woman? She has been treated "philanthropically"—Hegel long lauded Pinel for the humanity with which he approached the mad-women—but her mannerisms suggest that, despite this, she is no closer to being freed of her condition. Hysteria treatment under Charcot maintained this fluidity between the carnival and the clinical, but unlike Hegel and Pinel, Charcot always believed that he would find a lesion, a biological marker for hysteria, an authenticator of sorts. "Gentlemen, we have yet to determine the relationship that ought now to exist between pathology and physiology . . . the new physiology absolutely refuses to see life as a mysterious and supernatural influence, which acts as fancy takes it, free from all laws. Physiology goes so far as to believe that vital properties will one day be reduced to properties of a physical order."

Authenticity was at the core of all Charcot believed about hysteria, and during his medical seminars, spectacles in which he would hypnotize the hysteric and manipulate her attacks, he believed that the phenomenon of hypnosis was not the hallucination of a madwoman, insisting, rather, on the reality of the patient's perceptions. Blanche was questioned as to whether the hypnotized hysterics were faking it, to make fools of the doctors or the audience. "Simulation!" she exclaimed. "Do you think that it would have been easy to fool Monsieur Charcot? Oh yes, there were certainly some jokers who tried! He would look them straight in the eye and say 'Be still.'"

Recently, I edited a cluster of essays on the sociological, philosophical, literary, and personal interpretations of pain. In her essay, philosopher Jennifer Corns points out that pain is poorly correlated with pathology, and the subjective nature of patients' reports of pain complicates the treatment of pain alone: "As definitive of a medical condition, for use in clinical practice, a purely subjective definition is extraordinary. Imagine our surprise if the only accepted valid marker for any other medical condition, e.g., diabetes or cancer, was the subjective report. Imagine the absurdity of suggesting that the gold standard for diagnosing any other medical condition were patients' reports that they had it, or that the patient report was the only valid indicator of the condition." Corns's conclusion is that pain ought not be considered a treatment target and should, instead, be used as a jumping-off point for doctors to consider before investigating the underlying cause.

The assertion doesn't seem that radical, unless you have ever attempted to obtain treatment for, or investigate the underlying cause of, chronic pain—a long, expensive, usually fruitless process. I had many Behçet's symptoms for more than a decade before receiving a diagnosis. The American Auto-immune Related Diseases Association (AARDA) estimates that the average patient spends three years (and consults four doctors) before receiving an accurate diagnosis, and that some fifty million Americans have an autoimmune disease. Women experiencing chronic pain are more likely to be diagnosed with a mental disorder and prescribed psychotropic medication than they are to have their existing pain treated. Autoimmunity is an epidemic. Conditions without biomarkers or diagnostic tests, like fibromyalgia or myalgic encephalomyelitis (chronic fatigue syndrome), are further stigmatized and poorly understood. Most people haven't heard of my disease, but at least most doctors believe it's real. Even if I had never been diagnosed, I would still have the same symptoms. Idiopathic syndromes and conditions (that is, diseases of uncertain origin) often have testable abnormalities even when an organic cause cannot be found. That my abnormalities were not discovered despite a decade of concrete physical symptoms says less about what was going on with my body than it does about my not knowing which tests to ask for or when they needed to be conducted in order to provide useful results.

When I consider the immense difficulty of keeping myself alive through chronic illness—suffering through a decade of diagnostics, enduring miserable cycles of treatments, going into medical debt, working several jobs in order to maintain health insurance and be able to pay for it, and being subjected to everyday medical bureaucracy—I am overwhelmed by how much worse these multilayered cruelties are for patients who do not have the benefit of presenting as I do. My presentation to the medical gaze is mitigated by my whiteness. I am able to "pass" as healthy in everyday life, and the disease I was eventually diagnosed with is generally considered to be biological—which is to say, devoid of stigma or blame. All things considered, I should have had an easier time of things than many—particularly people of color, who are routinely undertreated and insufficiently anesthetized. While the concern of pharmacists and doctors about the addictive qualities of opiates are warranted, I wish that the sheer magnitude of the epidemic of chronic pain from all its possible sources warranted their similar concern.

Assertions that we should not consider ostensibly sourceless pain to be a worthy focus of treatment leads to an overemphasis of biology's role in legitimizing illness. It's the same kind of assumption that Charcot initially made—that all symptoms would eventually be traced back to some sort of biomarker. Sometimes, the assumption is correct: In his 1893 obituary for Charcot, Freud explained that the neurologist had employed a servant with a tremor disorder, despite how "in the course of the years she cost him a small fortune in dishes and plates," because he wanted to observe the anatomical basis for the tremor after her death. "When at last she died, he was able to demonstrate from her case that *paralysie choréiforme* was the clinical expression of multiple cerebro-spinal sclerosis." Charcot also successfully decoded the defining features of both multiple sclerosis and tabes dorsalis (the corrupted nerve function later known to be caused by syphilis). Other times, evidence of the biological nature of a condition is emphasized with the virtuous intention of getting suffering people treatment—as with Charcot's advocacy for the traumatized industrial workers. While the impetus to present conditions without observable organic cause or biomarkers as biological is often motivated by the desire to legitimize patients' real suffering, it also reinforces the problematic thinking that non-biologic illness is somehow unreal, illegitimate, or the result of a patient's laziness, lack of willpower, or choices.

We may one day know of a biologic cause for autoimmunity or other poorly understood conditions too easily relegated to the psychological, like myalgic encephalomyelitis or fibromyalgia. Nevertheless, current patients should be able to receive treatment to alleviate their systems without having to wait for biological vindication. The stakes are high: when conditions without known biomarkers present as culturally literate (that is, easily relegated to the realm of metaphor), this not only works against medical belief, but also informs how those conditions are treated. *Ill Feelings*, a striking memoir by Alice Hattrick about chronic fatigue syndrome (ME/CFS), one of the physically unexplained conditions often juxtaposed with hysteria, charts this phenomenon: "Medical diagnoses reflect societal ideas of what causes ill feelings, which is to say that, as a 'physically unexplained' syndrome, ME/CFS came to be considered, in the words of Simon Wessely, professor of psychological medicine at King's College, London, 'not simply an illness, but a cultural phenomenon and metaphor for our times.'" Wessely, who has influenced UK public health guidelines for ME/CFS and disability benefit revision, has pushed for a treatment program "focused on altering patients' belief that 'physical symptoms always imply tissue damage,' otherwise known as 'catastrophizing,' symptom focusing or 'bodywatching,' and 'behavioral factors such as persistent avoidance of activities associated with an increase in symptoms.'" In other words, treatment consists of trying to convince patients that their symptoms do not reveal anything about the physical reality of their bodies and instructing them to push through activities they understand to worsen their symptoms. If a patient's condition is chronic, and they remain unable to work—that is, to cure themselves *through* work—it can be read as their choice to resist treatment, to indulge their sick personality. This kind of contemporary account does not even dignify the sufferer with a label like the one Janet used for hysteria, a "malady through representation," with symptoms announcing what otherwise cannot be represented.

What people call the sick role is actually a result of the repeated blows of disbelief and abstraction patients face at every juncture in the diagnostic and treatment processes. No one experiences their own debilitating illness as metaphor, a problem of belief.

This is not to mention the myriad conditions that use the patient's subjective report as the only diagnostic measure for prescribing medication—like depression. SSRIs are routinely prescribed to people without the need for a specific diagnosis, and because depression treatment has capitalized on an unproven biological label, relegating ambiguously ill or autoimmune patients to psychiatric treatment is easier than ever. I've lost count of how many times—before, during, and even after my diagnosis of Behçet's—doctors suggested SSRIs to me, even while noting how "composed" I managed to be through all this. Before being diagnosed, I suffered exactly as I do now. I had the same symptoms. When I consulted neurologists for fainting spells, symptoms I now understand to have been caused by neuro-Behçet's were attributed to unstated feelings, depression, and anxiety. I was told that I did not even need to be aware that I was experiencing these feelings in order to be diagnosed with their corresponding disorders or for doctors to determine that they were what caused me to lose consciousness—all while the physical impact of my disease ran unchecked. It is unfortunate that the lasting impact of Freud's work in hysteria has been to predispose medical doctors to attribute mental states to patients that we often do not possess.

After my Behçet's diagnosis, my first rheumatologist tried to convince me again to try SSRIs; it was inconceivable to him that this painful and exhausting disease would make me feel anything but despondence. He wasn't wrong: despondence is often all I can feel. I have had major depressive episodes in concert with poor health my entire life. Those feelings are a response to my circumstances, not the toxic result of my own thoughts (as cognitive behavioral therapy, or CBT, posits) or a brain disease. It is conceivable that antidepressants would have made me feel better about the hopelessness of my bodily situation. Maybe they make many people with or without specific diagnoses feel better, but in none of those cases is a disease with objective, biological, data-specific qualities a prerequisite for medication. So, why is the treatment of physical pain continually up for debate?

Neuroscientist Anne Harrington provides some illuminating context. In *Mind Fixers: Psychiatry's Troubled Search for the Biology of Mental Illness*, she charts the distaste for psychoanalysis in favor of CBT and biological medical models as tied to a mythical 1980s "biological revolution" that didn't have as much to do with medical discovery as with a shift in public thought. Psychiatry presumes our brains to be already diseased; CBT presumes our thoughts to be already diseased. While psychoanalysis emerged in reaction to a biological focus in psychiatry, it also left "a generation of scapegoated parents" supposedly responsible for the mental unwellness of their children. To these parents, a return to a biological approach seemed like "a road to redemption," though Harrington argues that it also "overreached, overpromised, overdiagnosed, over-medicated" patients and "compromised" the field's principles.

If medicine, treatment for depression, addiction, and psychotherapy understood suffering to be inherently legitimate and worthy of specific and effective treatment, instead of acquiescing to an unproven biological label in order to get patients access to a less specific and possibly incorrect treatment, diagnostics might be more specific and useful, and patients could spend less time trying to convince their practitioners that our experiences don't line up with their classifications. Harrington's observation that biological psychiatric theories have a way of affixing themselves to an era's problematic beliefs about race or sex, while professing to be more humane than whatever came before, is particularly apt when considering Charcot's effort to destigmatize hysteria by classifying it as biological. (Though this goes both ways, as some of medicine's most horrific, torturous practices have been enacted in the search for a probable cause for biological distinctions between races.)

I do not cite Harrington's argument to suggest that mental disorders should not be treated as conditions—though she is particularly articulate in her debunking of the "chemical imbalance" and "bad wiring" narratives that are so ingrained in our culture they seem to be supported by considerably more science than they actually are—but to make the point that diagnosing an illness as biological *or* psychosomatic is often a way of obscuring the nature of the illness to the patient and offloading responsibility onto them, instead of making our society more livable for all kinds of sick and suffering people. A fainting girl can be told it's all in her head and sent to a psychiatrist, who will be unable to address the symptom, just as the depressed patient can be told they are unhappy due to a chemical imbalance and given medication in lieu of treatment that addresses, or at least considers, their personal circumstances or larger structural forces. Western medicine remains devastatingly attached to the notion of blame, to the extent that it is difficult even to critique the medical model without resorting to it.

To be depressed under late capitalism, as a result of physical illness or alienation, seems to me a rational response to one's conditions. However, when it prevents one from producing value through labor, it is considered an illness. Because of the way we have organized our society, the person who seeks treatment through submission to the medical gaze is a consumer; health is a kind of property, a sort of capital that can be used to generate more capital. In *Capitalist Realism*, Mark Fisher warns that "considering mental illness an individual chemico-biological problem has enormous benefits for capitalism"; the same can be said for the epidemic of autoimmunity. We cannot yet know the extent to which autoimmunity is a result of unchecked capitalist production and its runoff—Behçet's is correlated with, but not in requirement of, a gene and seems to be more common along Silk Road trade routes—but if we consider autoimmunity to be the conclusion of a medical and pharmaceutical model, recognized and treated according to a protocol, those who have not yet been diagnosed are simply bodies not yet capitalized by the pharma-consumer model. Without the medical-diagnostic industrial complex—the only real means of accessing potentially effective care in the United States—these diseases and the people who suffer from them do not exist. Bodies that fail under the conditions of capitalism get pathologized. The project of seeking diagnosis is an attempt at rectifying and recognizing pain that has often long been received with indifference. It can be eternally futile or eternally "successful" in that you never stop accruing diagnoses.

In order to monitor the inflammatory effects of my disease and my many medications, I have blood work done frequently. Many years into my treatment for Behçet's, my blood tests showed that I also have Sjogren's (an immune syndrome that impacts tear and saliva glands, frequently comorbid with other immune disorders), and likely also lupus. When I asked my rheumatologist if this last illness would change anything about how we were treating my Behçet's, she said it would not. I've also been told I have Raynaud's, a phenomenon of decreased blood flow to the fingers due to blood vessel spasm, but it is not clear if this is distinct from a similar manifestation of blood vessel action as a result of Behçet's. A criterion is useful for diagnosis only if it includes as many people who have the disease as possible, excludes those who do not, and describes symptoms as they appear in a medical setting. The more subjective the symptom appears clinically, the more likely it is to overlap with other conditions (that is, extremely likely, as is the case with autoimmune disease, depression, etc.).

Eli Clare, one of the first scholars to popularize the body-mind concept (in which the body and mind are expressed as a single, integrated unit), writes that diagnosis is "a tool and a weapon shaped by particular belief systems, useful and dangerous by turns"; that he wants "to read diagnosis as a source of knowledge, sometimes trustworthy and other times suspect." Diagnosis does not tell us much about the world, about the cruelty and indifference of medicine. It does not counteract punitive illness metaphors. It doesn't tell someone what their pain feels like or why a week in bed is the "price" of a fun night. Diagnosis does not stop you from resorting to blame and self-recrimination when you are faced with all the things you want to do but cannot do any longer. The impact of what diagnosis indicates falls outside the scope of what is considered medical. Behçet's is the name of a body that is not trusted, the name of a body that does not trust itself. Behçet's is lost ability. Behçet's is lost time. Behçet's is disappearance. Behçet's is experiencing moments of pleasure as future pain. Behçet's is the inability to untangle which experience of haziness comes from illness or medication. Behçet's is your mother saying, when you have nothing to report on the phone but suffering, that she *just can't believe* that you have this. Behçet's is a lover telling you he knows someone who cured their psoriasis through diet and that he doesn't see why you won't at least try the same. Behçet's is the room spinning through a meeting that could have been an email. Behçet's is spending months at a time with flu symptoms because your department has a policy that teachers should fail any student who does not attend 90 percent of class meetings, so students come to class sick. Behçet's is a job making you sick but also you needing the job so you can keep your health insurance to treat Behçet's. Behçet's is unpaid labor. Behçet's is the university proving, overnight, that online teaching—the kind of accommodation not previously offered as *reasonable*—is actually quite reasonable once able-bodied teachers are subject to risk as well. Behçet's is the adjunctification of universities. Behçet's is reapplying for your job each year under hiring practices that leave you afraid to present any reason for their not keeping you around. Behçet's is telling a sick student which blood tests she should ask for—the blood tests that might have gotten *you* a diagnosis a decade sooner.

Behçet's is a lifetime of student loan payments to cover the ambulance rides you took in college. Behçet's is recognizing which students are struggling physically or are fatigued from working night shifts. Behçet's is moving into an apartment you cannot afford when your roommate gets breast cancer in her thirties and your doctor advises against two people on the same immune suppressants living under one roof: *You'll both always be sick*. Behçet's is no CDC pandemic guidelines for the immune-compromised, even after a study of those with suppressed immune systems shows that only 17 percent had detectable antibodies after a Covid-19 vaccination. Behçet's is the CDC finally reporting, months later, that the vaccine may not be effective in people with suppressed immune systems, who should talk to their doctors and possibly continue to quarantine indefinitely. Behçet's is the CDC reporting that immune-suppressed people are not only more vulnerable to breakthrough infection, but also more likely to be vectors of infection for healthy people. Behçet's is a national pandemic "health" response not once decoupled from the economy. Behçet's is the single silver lining of the pandemic: being spared the constant contagion of unventilated classrooms full of undergraduates. Behçet's is taking an opiate in order to complete a wellness webinar. Behçet's is being told you might feel less fatigued by doing more. Behçet's is explaining what a cytokine storm is. Behçet's is saying that the idea of a "natural" treatment is nice but that your organs no longer function "naturally" and that for white patients to think of herbal and Eastern medicines as something more primitive, something they can just pick up and tune their bodies to, is rather epistemologically racist, actually. Behçet's is friendships lost to your inability to show up, lovers lost to their missed STD tests—for which you can't blame them, really, as you have so little to offer and don't want them around your brokenness. Behçet's is being able to tell only fundamentally ungracious stories. Behçet's is falling in love and learning to allow someone around your brokenness. Behçet's is shaving off bits of your soul. Behçet's is telling people it's a lot like lupus. Behçet's is something better described as being allergic to the entire world. Behçet's is something better described still as feeling so bad so much of the time that your real fear is that, soon, no high will pull you out of it. Behçet's is knowing you are totally and completely fucked, that your life force will continue to fractionalize, that pleasing people or having a career must slump away if you are ever to be able to write. Behçet's is reminding yourself, every day, even from bed, that you are one of the lucky ones.

The Cartesian binary describes the body in mechanical terms. Sontag references the oft-employed metaphor of the body "as a factory, an image of the body's functioning under the sign of health." In this conception, the chronically sick body, unable or unwilling to function as a factory, is in revolt. The James family frequently used economic metaphors in which one family member's health came at the "cost" of another's illness. Henry wrote of "a theory that this degenerescence of mine is the result of Alice and Willy getting better and locating some of their diseases on me." Did he really believe that one sibling's health could cause the others' pain? Such economic metaphors are some of the easiest to grasp toward when trying to explain to a healthy person how the basic expenditures of energy for everyday life seem to "cost" me more.

When I began the symptom diary that turned into writing projects that turned into this book, I worried about brain damage, memory loss, loss of my words. I wasn't sure which parts of me could be lost—to damage, to the dulling effects of lifesaving (or -prolonging) medications. Orienting myself toward whatever gave me the disease seemed a dead end, compared with trying to document the disease's impact on my relationship to the rest of the world or to investigate what, exactly, it may have taken from me.

While I have lived through a fairly constant tide of physical impairment, I have only recently become acclimated to referring to myself as "disabled." Disability is constructed against a capitalist ideal of ability. Unsurprisingly, my coming around to the term was not the result of revelation or self-understanding, but of having to navigate both the astounding lack of medical resources available for people who must work through chronic illness and workplaces not built with sick people in mind. I chose academic labor because it would allow me to structure more of my time than a nine-to-five and because I am not consistently capable of working forty-hour weeks sitting in a chair at an office. In academia, some of my work can be done from bed. (The Covid-19 pandemic quickly revealed that much more of it can be done from bed than our employers like to pretend is the case.) Each academic job application gives the federal ADA disclaimer, something along the lines of *Federal law requires employers to provide reasonable accommodation to qualified individuals with disabilities. Please tell us if you require reasonable accommodation to apply for a job or to perform your job. Examples of reasonable accommodation include making a change to the application process or work procedures, providing documents in an alternative format, using a sign language interpreter, or using specialized equipment.*

The perceived risk of disclosing a disability is contextual: chronic illness and its corresponding brain fog and cognitive decline are likely to be interpreted as a candidate's being unqualified. There are no alternative document formats or specialized equipment that will make working through pain and exhaustion more bearable. True accommodation would mean universal health care, a living wage that covers housing and nutritious food, debt forgiveness, sufficient time to rest, sick people being supported without fear of losing their jobs, and the abolition of all wellness webinars. As disabled poet Liz Bowen, in the previously mentioned cluster of essays I edited, wrote of her experience working through life-threatening illness to meet the demands of the academic job market, "We can theorize all we want about the breakdown of the mind-body divide, but if our labor practices don't allow for rest and healing, the critical thinking we are tasked with teaching others is a corrupt and empty enterprise."

A medical model of disability considers a person to be disabled by an impairing characteristic; a social model of disability defines the disabled not necessarily by something they lack but by society's *lack of accounting for them*. American disability activist Marta Russell moved beyond these two models and toward a Marxist materialist analysis of disability, considering what the systems of production extracted from the disabled. Quoting Russell, Beatrice Adler-Bolton and Artie Vierkant write in *Health Communism*:

> Under the money model of disability, "the disabled human being is a commodity around which social policies are created or rejected based on their market value." Russell argued that this constituted much more than simply profiting from the provision of medical care to the disabled. For Russell, the money model is presented as a corporate

"solution" to the problem of disablement, predicated on the primary assumption that "Disabled people are 'worth' more to the Gross Domestic Product when we occupy a 'bed' instead of a home . . . The 'final solution'—corporate dominion over disability policy—measures a person's 'worth' by its dollar value to the economy." The money model of disability identifies what is in essence a "cure" for the existence of unproductive bodies under capitalism.

Everyone is either sick or will become so. The brutality that health-as-capital commits forces us to "cease to be soldiers in the army of the upright," as Virginia Woolf put it—we "become deserters." The old adage that socialism never took root in America because the poor see themselves not as an exploited proletariat but as temporarily embarrassed millionaires seems to apply to health, too: only a people delusional that they will always be healthy and available for work could believe our capitalist arrangement of society to be anything but tyrannical, hateful, and targetedly cruel to the ill. As Russell puts it, "people with disabilities function as canaries in the coal mine" for what healthy workers can expect with the progression of capitalism. Yet, it is easy to erase the sites where illness occurs outside the workplace (hospitals, clinics, asylums, and the home) as those of political struggle. Foucault analyzed the conversion of leper management into plague management: lepers had been treated with exclusion from social life outside the community, while early modern plague management brought a more disciplinary approach, relegating bodies to confinement in homes. Where we put the sick determines what political action might look like and what we mean when we talk about "visibility."

The Socialist Patients' Collective (SPK), a West German organization of patients and doctor allies founded in 1970, thought illness was both the condition and the result of capitalism, the group's ethos summated in the slogan "Turn illness into a weapon." By reframing illness as a contradiction created by capitalism—and health as a "biological fascist fantasy"—the SPK held the conditions that the sick must live under accountable for their suffering, as opposed to treating suffering as an inevitability of biology. Their project of unifying and mobilizing the "sick proletariat" has been largely lost to history. The most comprehensive history of the group published in English can be found in Adler-Bolton and Vierkant's *Health Communism*. They write, "Unlike other self-organized patient groups and their counterparts in the anti-psychiatry movement, SPK uniquely combined Marxist political theory, social science analysis, and what they termed 'therapeutic praxis' to create an improvised, in-patient community with the express collectivist goal of researching the connections between capitalism, madness, eugenics, and the individuation of illness under political economies of work and care." As I began writing this book in graduate school, lines from the group's manifesto littered my desk:

> Subjectively the sick person is compelled
> through his or her suffering to make his existence,
> his life, the object of his consciousness.

Illness is inseparably bound up with
psychological stress, with the need for change,
with the need for production.

The success of the "treatment" gets
reified in the reproduction of the sick person's
employability, of their ability to function in the
anti-human, illness-engendering social production
process of capital, in their "rehabilitation."

Anyone can become acutely ill, all
are potential patients.

I cannot consider my illness outside a framework of cost. As a teenager, I thought illness and injury were the "cost" of ballet—to me, it seemed that transcendence and performance would require physical sacrifice. Balletic practice is also fraught with dualities—man/woman, good/evil—without which the notion of balletic beauty might crumble. New York City Ballet founding partner Lincoln Kirstein wrote in his 1984 essay "Beliefs of a Master" that ballet dancers must strive to be otherworldly and that "Balanchine's ballets can be read as icons for the laity, should we grant dancers attributes of earthly angels":

Modern and now postmodern dancers convince themselves and their annotators that minimal motion is as interesting to watch as to perform, at least to cult or coterie audiences in minimal spaces, clubs for companionship rather than frames for absolute skill. Minimal movement exploits a token idiom of natural motion: walk, turn, hop, run. Also, there is free-fall to the floor plus rolling and writhing. But angels don't jerk or twitch, except for irony or accent: they seem to swim or fly . . . Angels are androgynous, lacking heavy bosoms and buttocks. Portraits of angels in mural or mosaic have slight physiognomic distinction one from another. There is a blessed lack of "personality" in their stance against the skies. But this aerial or ethereal positioning grants them a special grace or magic in accepted service. Ballerinas are kin to those mythic Amazons who sliced off a breast to shoot arrows the more efficiently.

Trying to explain the appeal of ballet means resorting to such mythology and abstraction.

Balanchine positioned women as muses: "Ballet is woman," he famously proclaimed. "God made men to sing the praises of women. They aren't equal to men; they are better." Indeed, what makes Balanchine's choreography so magical is the agency with which the female roles are danced. The women are powerful, beautiful, larger-than-life muses whom men admire and serve. The appeal is not unlike the wordless tales told by the photographs of the hysterics. So often, the idealization of women acts as a means of their diminishment.

The impeachable character of the genius male artist is among the most prevalent motifs in ballet mythology, alongside the notion that serving ballet (for a woman) means refuting real life—forgoing health, higher education, financial stability, a social life, love, family. These sacrifices do not seem natural to me now; they seem like egregious labor issues. In the classic 1948 dance film *The Red Shoes*, Lermontov, the company impresario, warns, "A dancer who relies upon the doubtful comforts of human love will never be a great dancer—never." Vicky, his star dancer, falls in love with another dancer, Julian, and keeps their relationship a secret from Lermontov. No matter: Lermontov learns of the partnership and fires Julian, and Vicky leaves the company with him. When Lermontov coerces her back for a revival performance, both men contend for her, and she is caught between her love for Julian and her need to dance. She chooses the latter, and serving Lermontov is conflated with serving ballet itself. Loss of love is but another "cost" of dance, and the "balletic male genius's" mistreatment of female dancers only adds to the mystique surrounding him.

When I first met my friend Toni Bentley, a former Balanchine dancer turned writer, she showed me her right hip bone rolling around in a box hand-painted by Mr. B. himself, next to her last pair of pointe shoes; the bone had had to be replaced after she developed osteoarthritis in her early twenties, the cost of her labor. In 1982, Toni published a striking, unflinching memoir—the first tell-all of its kind in the American ballet world—of NYCB's winter 1980 season, when she was only twenty-two. Already she sensed that, despite her profound ambition and talent, her career might end right where she was: in the corps. *Winter Season: A Dancer's Journal* foretells the writer she would become—concerned with masochism, corporeality, impossible beauty, ruin, and release, her tendency to think too much to be a dancer. The book has been aptly lauded as a testament to the company, to Balanchine, and to the extreme lives of dancers. Kirstein wrote to Toni years later that she had written "the best book on our company, and . . . painted the best portrait of Balanchine that exists"—but it is also an incredible document of the labor issues of the era. In it, Toni documents the yearlong negotiations between NYCB management and the NYCB union, the American Guild of Musical Artists (AGMA). During this time, the dancers were working without a contract:

If a dancer speaks, it must have value. What I'm trying to say is that we are all grossly ignorant of money matters, our rights, and even what we can and should demand—but we try. We attempt to explain to these men our perverse and unique situation. We are under the dictatorship of one man, whom we adore and respect, and his every whim is our law, no questions asked.

A union? A democracy under a dictator? We have no power to strike, really. Who would do that to our god?

To negotiate the terms of one's contract was to negotiate the value of Balanchine himself. Balanchine guilted the dancers for the union's strike for a living wage, reminding them that he and his peers had slept on the floor as starving young dancers. Toni wrote that she felt "cheated of a time of suffering such as Mr. B. had. We have had no opportunity to starve and work and live on the edge. We starve ourselves only out of neurosis. We are spoiled."

Is it possible to untangle abjection and asceticism from labor? Even today, the commodification and exploitation of dancers is discussed mainly as an issue of emotional or physical abuse or the cult of personality, but surely one need not write off Balanchine as a Svengali in order to argue that the conditions of late capitalism dictate what kind of artistry is possible for choreographers and dancers, just as they dictate the kind of learning environment I am able to offer my students. McCarren, in *Dance Pathologies*, suggests that Marx's redefinition of physical labor as "physical expenditure" helped facilitate the disconnection of dance from Foucault's idea of *désœuvrement*: the absence of work that defined madness in the nineteenth century. Because dance is work and performance and art, it cannot be *désœuvrement*—according to Foucault, "Where there is a work of art, there is no madness."

Toni comes to think of her deprivation of a life outside the ballet world differently later in the book, in a passage written on her twenty-third birthday: "I think I've discovered my problem— not the cure, but the problem. It is not dancing that has been making me miserable, it is what dancing does not allow that I've missed . . . I am starved for people, life, thoughts, conversation, alternatives to my NYCB world. I need only a few hours out in the real world to return joyful and by choice to my tendus." Still, she suspected, her days in ballet were numbered. A few pages later, in a passage that could have been lifted from my despondent teenage diaries, she writes, "The eternal struggle—to give in to one's weakness, or disregard it and forge ahead. I've always chosen the second, and the weaknesses vanished. Now they have emerged stronger than ever."

In *The Red Shoes*, when Lermontov asks Vicky why she wants to dance, she responds by asking him, "Why do you want to live?" Now, revisiting the memoirs and autobiographies of the dancers I admired as a child, I notice that while most do not conceive of balletic labor as specifically as Toni—and all are in agreement that they do not dance only for a living but also to live—these women have certainly been warning one another of the cultural conditions of the ballet world all along. Like many young dancers, I devoured former NYCB principal Gelsey Kirkland's 1986 autobiography, *Dancing on My Grave*, which chronicles her rise from star student to principal dancer, her drug addiction and physical deterioration, and the pitfalls of being locked into Balanchine's closed system of instruction. I first read the book between classes in the crumbling building of my ballet school, breathing the characteristic scent of rosin, sweat, and Jet glue while the other girls stretched and tittered as the boys struggled to balance in their pointe shoes. For many, these interactions were their earliest flirtations, branded by the slightest betrayal of the strict balletic gender divide: women wear pointe shoes, extending their limbs to their most lengthened iteration; men lift the women up. Kirkland's suggestion that "ballet seemed infinitely preferable to the kind of romantic exchange valued by my peers" had deeply resonated with me: How could the other students see their childish dalliances as worthwhile when we were learning the highest, most soulful art form? If they had enough desire left over for anything else, did they really love ballet all that much? I think of this young girl often: how the ideals of ballet might create hardship when she gets around to untangling her sexuality from dance— if she is able to. My tattered copy of Kirkland's book is long lost, so I checked out a copy from the library. In the margin of one page, as if to prepare for an interview with the writer, a previous borrower had written: "Ask why she's so obsessed w/ him" (as though the book were not partially an attempt by Kirkland to figure this out for herself). Some of the book's most potent passages are when Kirkland recalls objectifying Balanchine, perhaps because they are the sole moments when believing in his magic does not come at her expense: "I developed the habit of mentally undressing him, without any attraction, simply fascinated to know if he possessed all the attributes of the male anatomy. In an effort to rationalize the idle speculation about his sexual inadequacy, I told myself that when God gave out genius, the other areas might be slighted, like a blessing withheld. I never considered the possibility that Balanchine's genius and sexuality might be aberrations."

The line between the male genius (Toni Bentley's Balanchine, whom I am admittedly partial to) and the tyrant (Gelsey Kirkland's Balanchine) is seldom clear. Contemporary depictions of Doctor Charcot often depict him somewhere between a sexist, authoritarian sadist who slept with his patients and someone a bit too keen to document the hysterics' fantastically visual, sexualized symptoms. Swedish doctor and psychiatrist Axel Munthe, who had been a medical student of Charcot's, writes in his autobiographical novel, *The Story of San Michele*, about Charcot's methods as fraudulent and scientifically unsound. Munthe's hostility toward Charcot likely originated from an incident in which Munthe helped a patient escape from the ward of the hospital and brought her to his home. Charcot threatened to report him to the police and said that he would not be allowed in the Salpêtrière again.

The story reveals little about Charcot's true nature. What it does reveal is that some of the women did not believe that the treatments offered at the Salpêtrière were helping their condition. Some of them surely refused to be hypnotized, as Augustine had. Some of them desperately wanted to leave.

It is the second spring consumed by the Covid-19 pandemic. I am supposed to be at work on my memoir. That is what I have sold this book as: a memoir. In some sense, it is a relief. Autobiographical writing's sustaining fiction—that the writer and the subject are a cohesive, singular entity—can now be, explicitly, my object of contemplation. In another sense, it is bewildering: in graduate school, my work tended to be read as personal even when I was abstracting or writing in the third person. While I try not to get hung up on distinctions that are inconsequential outside the scope of book marketing, I know that if I am to offer an account undeniably of myself, it ought to be coherent, worthy of consideration—yet, my sense of a coherent self has been marred. Illness lends a certain understanding of this fragmentation of the observing/observed self.

The publisher's announcement of this book's future release describes it as "a memoir of revelation through chronic pain."

But I don't think pain is revelatory, I complained to a friend upon reading this. *I don't think my pain has taught me anything.*

When someone suggests that surely there are lessons or positives to be taken away from pain and suffering, it sounds as tone-deaf as the unsolicited suggestions of diets or healers—a vain, human effort to ascribe meaning when there is none.

Such suggestions usually come from the sort of optimist who seeks to make the pain of witness more bearable, who cannot stand the reality not only that chronic illness can seldom be triumphed over, but also that it does not necessarily teach us anything or help us grow. My worst self is the embodied result of pain and suffering. If someone is telling you their cautionary tale, it means that caution was not heeded. In the case of illness, it can't be: if you are young and well, you will not be so indefinitely, and there is nothing I can write to relieve a future sufferer of anxiety toward a future illness. There will be no lessons or imparted wisdom. It will not be worth it. The fundamental ungraciousness of choosing to tell this story—a story from which the only "wisdom" to be gleaned is a knowledge both structural and personal of the hell our capitalist arrangement of the world creates for the sick—is not lost on me.

Nevertheless, I want a painful clarity of illness. I want to prioritize concrete detail over abstraction, to reject that a story of endurance can be granted resolution. Unwavering commitment to the truth in the face of plummeting corporeal possibility is nearly impossible. Susan Sontag's son, David Rieff, wrote that, in her final days of treatment for myelodysplastic syndromes (MDS), his mother seemed to need "to find a way to look away and yet to feel as if she were not looking away, that it was an impossible balancing act. For it was as if she were trying to remain loyal to the idea of the truth and to the supremacy of the factual yet at the same time looking for ways to deny what these facts suggested." How we feel we ought to act in the face of immense pain and what we are capable of are seldom aligned. Rieff recalls reading one of

Sontag's journal entries, written after her breast cancer surgery years prior: "Despair shall set you free." He initially assumed his mother was making a morbid joke, but she continues entirely in earnest: "I can't write because I don't (won't) give myself permission to voice the despair I feel. Always the will. My refusal of despair is blocking my energies."

"I lived on a high horse," Sontag writes in another entry, "without saddle sores."

I live on a high horse with all kinds of sores.

Writing this book has been an exercise in submission to that despair; to my evisceration; to my unsaved life; to form imposed on an array of obsessions, premonitions, desires. I have kept Augustine's photos before me as I write. They can tell me nothing about how to approach the mind-body problem, do not translate intellectual principles into visceral ones, do not grant language to pain. They show me nothing but a woman at a moment in time. I have attempted to capture how she, through images of her body, which was subjected to a cruel and violent world, has affected my life.

Even the solace provided in hospital life under Charcot, Augustine's initial yes was eventually unendurable. We don't know what anything felt like for her after she left the Salpêtrière, if she was able to confront the soulful perils of the world she previously could not endure. We have no idea what happened to her next.

Finding the right words is paramount. The "language" hysteria provided to Augustine was ultimately insufficient, and playing the role of the model hysteric, the medical pin-up girl, became more oppressive than her symptoms. After refusing Charcot's hypnotism sessions, Augustine was placed in solitary confinement and gave a final expression of distress: the last entry in her medical file reads, "On September 9, Augustine escaped from the Salpêtrière, disguised as a man."

ACKNOWLEDGMENTS

Thank you to my professors and fellow students in the fiction workshop at UC Riverside for their early encouragement to pursue this story. Thanks in particular to my mentors, Charmaine Craig and Andrew Winer, whose nurturing care has fundamentally shaped me as a writer and person. I am grateful for expansive literary conversations with friends, especially Kamala Puligandla, Toni Bentley, and William J. Simmons.

I also wish to thank my wise editors, Lauren Hooker and Oona Holahan, and the entire team at Seven Stories. For his intrepid belief in this project, I owe tremendous gratitude to my agent, Jon Curzon. This is a book about living with literature, and I am indebted to the many writers who have provided source material and illuminated my life. Thanks to my parents and post-diagnosis doctors for keeping me alive. I also appreciate the nurses, lab technicians, administrative workers, and others whose labor has made my care possible.

Thanks most of all to Aaron Bornstein for our life, in sickness and in health.

SOURCES

Epigraph: "Be very careful not to understand the patient": Jacques Lacan, *The Ego in Freud's Theory and in the Technique of Psychoanalysis*, 1954–1955 (New York; London: W.W. Norton & Company, 1991), 2:87.

11   "I inscribe what I see": Georges Didi-Huberman, *Invention of Hysteria: Charcot and the Photographic Iconography of the Salpêtrière* (Cambridge, MA: MIT Press, 2003), 29.

11   "the true retina of the scientist": Didi-Huberman, *Invention of Hysteria*, 32.

22   "express the most vivid interest in": Albert Smith, *The Natural History of the Ballet-girl* (London: Dance Books, 1996), 46.

23   "in a culture that views dancers as vaguely 'sick'": Felicia M. McCarren, *Dance Pathologies: Performance, Poetics, Medicine* (Stanford, CA: Stanford University Press, 1998), 14.

23   "a predominant role": Jean-Martin Charcot et al., *Les Démoniaques dans l'art* (Paris: Macula, 1984), 34.

24   "many of the nightmares": McCarren, *Dance Pathologies*, 70.

25   "the definition of hysteria has never been given": Laségue, quoted in Pierre Janet, *L'État mental des hystériques* (Marseille: Laffitte, 1983), 411.

25   "less linear than it is cyclical": Mark S. Micale, *Approaching Hysteria: Disease and Its Interpretations* (Princeton, NJ: Princeton University Press, 1995), 19–29.

25   "Charles Le Pois argued": *Approaching Hysteria: Disease and Its Interpretations* (Princeton, NJ: Princeton University Press, 1995), 21.

26   "British clinician": *Approaching Hysteria: Disease and Its Interpretations* (Princeton, NJ: Princeton University Press, 1995), 22.

26   "Ovarian theory": *Approaching Hysteria: Disease and Its Interpretations* (Princeton, NJ: Princeton University Press, 1995), 23.

27   "Freud's development of the practice of psychoanalysis": Micale, *Approaching Hysteria*, 27.

31   "Owing to some physical weakness": Alice James, ed. Leon Edel, *The Diary of Alice James* (New York: Dodd, Mead and Company, 1964), 148–50.

32   "abandons part of her consciousness": William James, "The Hidden Self," Wikisource, n.d., en.wikisource.org/wiki/The_Hidden_Self.

37   "All the efforts of pathological anatomy": Didi-Huberman, *Invention of Hysteria*, 71; James, *The Diary of Alice James* (Boston, MA: Northeastern University Press, 1999), 142.

38   "the hysteric always seems to be outside the rule": Asti Hustvedt, *Medical Muses: Hysteria in Nineteenth-Century Paris* (New York: W.W. Norton and Company, 2011), 21.

38   One of them, Marie "Blanche" Wittman: Hustvedt, *Medical Muses*, 46.

40   "That depends on what you mean": Quoted in Allan Ulrich, "Cullberg Ballet on the Cusp: A Change in Rep for the Swedish Company That's Had Mats Ek Written All over It," The Free Library, n.d., www.thefreelibrary.com/Cullberg+Ballet+on+the+-cusp%3a+a+change+in+rep+for+the+Swedish+company...-a092135999.

42   *Les Démoniaques dans l'art*: Cristina Mazzoni, *Saint Hysteria: Neurosis, Mysticism, and Gender in European Culture* (Ithaca, NY: Cornell University Press, 1996), 28.

43   "[Charcot] has set forth some nervous phenomena": Guy de Maupassant, *The Works of Guy de Maupassant: Short Stories* (Rockville, MD: Wildside Press, 2010), 516.

44   "that He was within me": Teresa of Avila and J M Cohen, *The Life of Saint Teresa of Avila* (London: Penguin Books, 1957), 71.

44   "A pandemic similar to the one we see today": Tiqqun, trans. Ariana Reines, *Preliminary Materials for a Theory of the Young-Girl* (Cambridge, MA: MIT Press, 2012), 123.

45   "culturally permissible expressions of distress": Elaine Showalter, *Hystories: Hysterical Epidemics and Modern Culture* (London: Picador, 1997), 15.

45   "Suffering is instructive": Alphonse Daudet, trans. Julian Barnes, *In the Land of Pain* (London: Jonathan Cape, 2002), 3.

46   "Poor Daudet, who is haunted": Julien Bogousslavsky, *Neurological Disorders in Famous Artists* (Basel; Freiburgbreisgau: Karger, 2005), 41.

48   "Hysterics suffer for the most part from reminiscences": Sigmund Freud, Josef Breuer, and Nicola Luckhurst, *Studies in Hysteria* (New York: Penguin Books, 2004), 11.

50   "a mechanism which in the first instance": Talcott Parsons, *The Social System* (London: Routledge and Kegan Paul, 1951), 477.

52   "To understand this one painting": Allan H. Ropper and Brian Burrell, *How the Brain Lost Its Mind: Sex, Hysteria, and the Riddle of Mental Illness* (New York: Avery/Penguin Random House, 2019), 11.

53   "Everything in her": Désiré Bourneville and Paul Regnard, *Iconographie photographique de la Salpêtrière* (Paris: Progrès médical, 1878), 2:168, quoted in Hustvedt *Medical Muses*, 169.

60   "We must say that we regret": *British Medical Journal* (London: British Medical Association, 1879), 857.

62   "pulled her hair, tickled, punched": Hustvedt, *Medical Muses*, 169.

62   "Before the[ir] attacks": Y. Keydar, "Mysteria: Unraveling Hysteria Theory Through Mid- to Late-Nineteenth-Century Fashion," (*History of Costume 2*, term paper, MA Costume Studies Program, NYU Steinhardt, 2015)..

62 "Both in the admission reports": Maayan Goldman, "Dressing like a Madwoman: On Amanda Bynes, Little Edie, and the Time I Quite Fashion," Vestoj, n.d., vestoj. com/dressing-like-a-madwoman/.

66 "Here brought to Ballet is the atmosphere, or nothing": Stéphane Mallarmé, *Oeuvres complètes* (Paris: Pléiade, 1945), 313, quoted and translated in McCarren, *Dance Pathologies*, 117.

66 "hypnotism at that moment": Loie Fuller, *Fifteen Years of a Dancer's Life: With Some Account of Her Distinguished Friends* (London: H. Jenkins Limited, 1913), 25.

66 "I endeavoured to make myself as light": Fuller, *Fifteen Years of a Dancer's Life*, 31.

67 "Mallarmé's dance texts on Loie Fuller": McCarren, *Dance Pathologies*, 25.

67 "Mallarmé describes Fuller's performing persona": McCarren, *Dance Pathologies*, 157.

68 "functions as a critique of Charcotian psychology": McCarren, *Dance Pathologies*, 25.

71 "A doctor in Northern Germany": Twitter user @jtheseamstress, Twitter post, February 2019, 10:26 p.m., twitter.com/jtheseamstress/status/1093395579584086016.

72 "The sufferings most often deemed worthy": Susan Sontag, *Regarding the Pain of Others* (New York: Farrar, Straus and Giroux, 2003), 40.

76 "examines the gender hierarchy": Rachel Mesch, *The Hysteric's Revenge: French Women Writers at the Fin de Siècle* (Nashville, TN: Vanderbilt University Press, 2006), 129.

77 "Dissatisfaction is the motor for desire": Anouchka Grose, introduction to *Hysteria Today* (Abingdon; New York: Routledge, 2018), xxx.

78 "literally cannot live or function": Louise Bourgeois's diary, quoted in Juliet Mitchell, "Louise Bourgeois and Sigmund Freud: Passage Dangereux—The Girl in Psychoanalysis and Art," in Louise Bourgeois et al., *Louise Bourgeois, Freud's Daughter* (New Haven, CT/London: Yale University Press, 2021), 137.

78 "Since the fears of the past": Louise Bourgeois, cited in "Self-expression Is Sacred and Fatal," in Christiane Meyer-Thoss, *Louise Bourgeois: Designing by Free Fall* (Zürich: Ink Press, 2016), 228.

80 "In Bourgeois's terms": Philip Larratt-Smith, "The Case of LB," in Bourgeois et al., *Louise Bourgeois, Freud's Daughter*, 107.

81 "The empty house": Louise Bourgeois's diary, quoted in Mitchell, "Louise Bourgeois and Sigmund Freud: Passage Dangereux—The Girl in Psychoanalysis and Art," 141.

81 "Bourgeois shows that": Juliet Mitchell, "Louise Bourgeois and Sigmund Freud: Passage Dangereux—The Girl in Psychoanalysis and Art," 139.

83 "rape, blood, more fires": Didi-Huberman, *Invention of Hysteria*, 137.

83 "when the men around her speak": Didi-Huberman, *Invention of Hysteria*, 137.

83 "vocalization, not communication": Hustvedt, *Medical Muses*, 188.

83 "You see how hysterics scream": Hustvedt, *Medical Muses*, 188–189.

84 "While it is not mentioned in the text": Hustvedt, *Medical Muses*, 153.

85 "A man like you, a forty year old man": Bourneville and Regnard, *Iconographie photographique de la Salpêtrière*, 2:161, quoted in Hustvedt, *Medical Muses*, 192.

85 "so that our readers can clearly appreciate": Bourneville and Regnard, *Iconographie photographique de la Salpêtrière*, 2:167, quoted in Hustvedt, *Medical Muses*, 194.

87 "He used to look": Freud, "Charcot" in *The Freud Reader*, 52, quoted in Hustvedt, *Medical Muses*, 21.

88 "In Agnes Varda's 1962 film": *Cléo from 5 to 7*, directed by Agnes Varda (Criterion Collection, 1962).

92 "For the sake of brevity": Sigmund Freud, Josef Breuer, and Nicola Luckhurst, *Studies in Hysteria* (New York: Penguin Books, 2004), 81.

93 "The problem with Charcot's work": Jacqueline Rose, "Femininity and Its Discontents," *Feminist Review* 14 (1983): 5–21.

94 "Is Hysteria Real? Brain Images Say Yes": Erika Kinetz, "Is Hysteria Real? Brain Images Say Yes," *New York Times*, September 26, 2006, www.nytimes.com/2006/09/26/science/26hysteria.html.

94 "demonstrate that there are neuroanatomical correlates": Siri Hustvedt, *The Shaking Woman, or, a History of My Nerves* (New York: Picador/Henry Holt, 2011), 34.

97 "Always the genital thing": Cristina Mazzoni, *Saint Hysteria: Neurosis, Mysticism, and Gender in European Culture* (Ithaca, NY: Cornell University Press, 1996), 21.

99 "The title assures me": Joanne Zeis, *You Are Not Alone: 15 People with Behçet's*, 1997.

99 "plenty of rest, maintain daily routine": Sungnack Lee et al., *Behçet's Disease: A Guide to Its Clinical Understanding Textbook and Atlas* (Berlin and Heidelberg: Springer Berlin Heidelberg, 2001), 73.

99 "Ever since I have been ill": James, *The Diary of Alice James* (New York edition), 206.

102 "Diagnosis has diminished my ability": Anne Boyer, *The Undying: Pain, Vulnerability, Mortality, Medicine, Art, Time, Dreams, Data, Exhaustion, Cancer . . . and Care* (New York: Picador, 2020), 35.

102 "A new language": Virginia Woolf, *On Being Ill* (1930; repr., Ashfield, MA: Paris Press, 2012), 7.

102 "lacked plot": Virginia Woolf, *On Being Ill* (1930; repr., Ashfield, MA: Paris Press, 2012), 6.

102 "we go alone": Virginia Woolf, *On Being Ill* (1930; repr., Ashfield, MA: Paris Press, 2012), 12.

103 "Suppose for a moment the claims": Anne Boyer, *The Undying*, 213.

103 "Contrast this philosophical truism": Anne Boyer, *The Undying*, 214.

104 "the pain [will] not be wasted": Audre Lorde, *The Cancer Journals* (London: Penguin Publishing Group, 2020), 9.

104 "But I think the only thing that could paralyze one's writing": Hélène Cixous and Susan Sellers, *White Ink: Interviews on Sex, Text, and Politics* (Hoboken, NJ: Taylor and Francis, 2014), 28.

104 "pain is always new to the sufferer": Daudet, *In the Land of Pain*, 19.

108 "told me he'd forgotten how completely the body loses": Hervé Guibert, *To the Friend Who Did Not Save My Life* (South Pasadena, CA: Semiotext(e), 2020), 36–37.

108 "the whole truth is still hidden from me": Guibert, *To the Friend Who Did Not Save My Life*, 17.

108 "already dead, beyond hope of salvation": Guibert, *To the Friend Who Did Not Save My Life*, 212.

108 "sleek and dazzling in its hideousness": Guibert, *To the Friend Who Did Not Save My Life*, 262.

108 "Between fits of coughing": Guibert, *To the Friend Who Did Not Save My Life*, 35.

109 "la belle indifference": Jon Stone et al., "La Belle Indifférence in Conversion Symptoms and Hysteria: Systematic Review," *The British Journal of Psychiatry: The Journal of Mental Science* 188 (2006): 204–9, https://doi.org/10.1192/bjp.188.3.204.

110 "take all the morphia": William James, *The Letters of William James* (Boston: Little, Brown, 1920), 311.

111 "My book is closing in on me": Guibert, *To the Friend Who Did Not Save My Life*, 251.

113 "Around her neck, she is wearing": W. G. Sebald, *Austerlitz* (London: Penguin, 2010), 350–51.

114 "For Barthes, the punctum": Roland Barthes, *Camera Lucida: Reflections on Photography* (New York: Hill And Wang, 1996), 27.

120 "Researchers will be studying": Dana Brandt and John Diedrich, "Nearly 800 People Have Died from Covid-19 in Wisconsin. Here's What We Are Learning so Far," *Journal Sentinel*, July 3, 2020, www.jsonline.com/story/news/2020/07/03/800-deaths-wisconsin-what-we-know-so-far-covid-19-coronavirus/5355666002/.

120 "the idea that any of the death and despair": Beatrice Adler-Bolton, "'Deaths Pulled from the Future,'" Blind Archive, January 3, 2022, blindarchive.substack.com/p/deaths-pulled-from-the-future.

121 "Derrida argued": Michael Naas, "'One Nation . . . Indivisible': Jacques Derrida on the Autoimmunity of Democracy and the Sovereignty of God," *Research in Phenomenology* 36, no. 1 (2006), https://doi.org/10.1163/156916406779165818.

121 "But you're not trying to want something else": Susan Sontag, *Alice in Bed: A Play* (New York: Farrer, Straus and Giroux, 1993), 20.

121 "I always thought a man would crush me": Sontag, *Alice in Bed*, 67.

122 "the religion of healthy-mindedness": Anne Harrington, *The Cure Within: A History of Mind-Body Medicine* (New York: W.W. Norton, 2008), 111.

122 "When I asked her what attitude of the mind": Alice James to William James, November 25, 1889, in *The Death and Letters of Alice James*, ed. Ruth Yeazell (Cambridge, MA: Exact Change, 2004), 181–82.

122 "As I lay prostrate": James, *The Diary of Alice James* (New York edition), 149.

123 "I shall at least have it all my own way": James, *The Diary of Alice James* (New York edition), 25.

134 stories of "night doctors" had circulated: Rebecca Skloot, *The Immortal Life of Henrietta Lacks* (New York: Broadway Books, 2010), 165–68.

136 "It is no accident": Benjamin quoted in Henry Bond, *Lacan at the Scene* (Cambridge, MA: MIT Press, 2012), 23.

137 "by practicing a social segregation": Michel Foucault, *Madness and Civilization: A History of Insanity in the Age of Reason* (New York: Vintage Books, 1973), 259.

139 "the grand asylum of human misery," "the living museum of pathology": Hustvedt, *Medical Muses*, 12.

144 "characterized by the subversion of the relationships": Louis Aragon and André Breton, "Le Cinquantenaire de l'hystérie," *La Révolution surréaliste*, March 15, 1928, 22, quoted in Mark S. Micale, *The Mind of Modernism: Medicine, Psychology, and the Cultural Arts in Europe and America* (Stanford, CA: Stanford University Press, 2004), 124.

144 "Beauty will be convulsive": André Breton, *Nadja* (New York: Grove Press, 1960), 160.

144 "the greatest poetic discovery": Micale, *The Mind of Modernism*, 124.

145 "It is also well to prepare": Emily Post quoted in Joan Didion, *The Year of Magical Thinking* (New York: Vintage Books, 2005), 59.

149 "Semmelweis dashed himself": Louis-Ferdinand Céline, *Semmelweis* (London: Atlas Press, 2008), 48.

150 "A reciprocity of charm was instituted": Didi-Huberman, *Invention of Hysteria*, xi.

150 Huberman adds that he is "nearly compelled": Didi-Huberman, *Invention of Hysteria*, 4.

151 "a simple contradiction within reason," "just as physical disease is not an abstract": Georg W. zf. Hegel, "Part III: The Philosophy of Spirit, (1830)," sec. 388, *Encyclopaedia of the Philosophical Sciences*, www.marxists.org, www.marxists.org/reference/archive/hegel/works/sp/susoul.htm.

151 "Gentlemen, we have yet to determine": Charcot, quoted in Didi-Huberman, *Invention of Hysteria*, 21.

152 "Do you think that it would have been easy": Hustvedt, *Medical Muses*, 141.

153 "As definitive of a medical condition": Jennifer Corns, "Puzzles with Pain Reports," Post45, February 24, 2020, post45.org/2020/02/puzzles-with-pain-reports/.

154 the average patient spends three years: Marie Benz, MD, FAAD, "Survey Finds Autoimmune Diseases Are Misunderstood, Common and Underfunded," October 3, 2018, https://medicalresearch.com/survey-finds-autoimmune-diseases-are-mis-understood-common-and-underfunded/

155 "in the course of the years she cost him a small fortune": Anne Harrington, *Mind Fixers: Psychiatry's Troubled Search for the Biology of Mental Illness* (New York: W.W. Norton, 2019), 12.

155 "when at last she died": Anne Harrington, *Mind Fixers: Psychiatry's Troubled Search for the Biology of Mental Illness* (New York: W.W. Norton, 2019), 12.

156 "Medical diagnoses reflect societal ideas": Alice Hattrick, *Ill Feelings* (London: Fitzcarraldo, 2021), 205.

156 "focused on altering": Alice Hattrick, *Ill Feelings* (London: Fitzcarraldo, 2021), 206.

157 "malady through representation": Pierre Janet, *The Mental State of Hystericals* (New York and London: Putnam, 1901), 486-8.

158 "biological revolution": Anne Harrington, *Mind Fixers: Psychiatry's Troubled Search for the Biology of Mental Illness* (New York: W.W. Norton & Company, 2019), xiv.

159 "a generation of scapegoated parents": Anne Harrington, *Mind Fixers: Psychiatry's Troubled Search for the Biology of Mental Illness* (New York: W.W. Norton & Company, 2019),181.

159 "a road to redemption": Anne Harrington, *Mind Fixers: Psychiatry's Troubled Search for the Biology of Mental Illness* (New York: W.W. Norton & Company, 2019),177.

159 "overreached, overpromised": Anne Harrington, *Mind Fixers: Psychiatry's Troubled Search for the Biology of Mental Illness* (New York: W.W. Norton & Company, 2019), xiv. 159 "considering mental illness an individual": Mark Fisher, *Capitalist Realism: Is There No Alternative?* (Winchester, UK: Zer0 Books, 2009), 37.

162 "a tool and a weapon shaped by particular belief systems": Eli Clare, *Brilliant Imperfection: Grappling with Cure* (Durham, NC: Duke University Press, 2017), 41.

165 "as a factory, an image of the body's functioning": Susan Sontag, *Illness as Metaphor and AIDS and Its Metaphors* (New York: Anchor Books, 1990), 96.

165 "a theory that this degenerescence": Henry James, *Selected Letters* (Cambridge, MA: Harvard University Press, 1987), 53.

167 "We can theorize all we want": Liz Bowen, "The Job Market Is Killing Me," Post45, February 24, 2020, https://post45.org/2020/02/the-job-market-is-killing-me/.

167 "Under the money model of disability": Beatrice Adler-Bolton and Artie Vierkant, *Health Communism* (London and Brooklyn, NY: Verso, 2022), 15.

168 "cease to be soldiers in the army of the upright": Virginia Woolf, "On Being Ill," *The Criterion*, 1926, thenewcriterion1926.files.wordpress.com/2014/12/woolf-on-being-ill.pdf.

168 "people with disabilities function as canaries": Marta Russell, *Beyond Ramps: Disability at the End of the Social Contract—A Warning from an Uppity Crip* (Monroe, ME: Common Courage Press, 1998), 98.

169 "Turn illness into a weapon": Socialist Patients' Collective, "Turn Illness into a Weapon: A Polemic Call for Action," Heidelberg University, www.indybay.org/uploads/2013/11/14/turn_illness_into_a_weapon.pdf.

169 "Unlike other self-organized patient groups": Adler-Bolton and Vierkant, *Health Communism*, 129.

171 "Balanchine's ballets can be read as icons": Lincoln Kirstein, "Beliefs of a Master: Lincoln Kirstein," *New York Review*, March 15, 1984, https://www.nybooks.com/articles/1984/03/15/beliefs-of-a-master/.

172 "Ballet is woman": Alastair Macaulay, "Of Women, Men and Ballet in the 21st Century," *The New York Times*, January 12, 2017, https://www.nytimes.com/2017/01/12/arts/dance/of-women-men-and-ballet-in-the-21st-century.html.

172 "God made men": "Harry Hurt III, "Paper Balanchine," *The New York Times*, March 10, 2007, sec. Business, https://www.nytimes.com/2007/03/10/business/10pursuits.ready.html.

174 "If a dancer speaks, it must have value": Toni Bentley, *Winter Season: A Dancer's Journal* (Gainesville: University Press of Florida, 2003), 33.

174 "cheated of a time of suffering": Bentley, *Winter Season*, 91.

175 "Where there is a work of art, there is no madness": Michel Foucault, *Madness and Civilization*, quoted in McCarren, *Dance Pathologies*, 37.

175 "I think I've discovered my problem": Bentley, *Winter Season*, 117.

175 "The eternal struggle": Bentley, *Winter Season*, 120.

176 "ballet seemed infinitely preferable": Gelsey Kirkland, *Dancing on my Grave: An Autobiography* (Garden City, NY: Doubleday & Company, 1986), 41.

176 "I developed the habit of mentally undressing him": Gelsey Kirkland, *Dancing on my Grave: An Autobiography* (Garden City, NY: Doubleday & Company, 1986), 50.

179 "to find a way to look away and yet to feel": David Rieff, *Swimming in a Sea of Death: A Son's Memoir* (New York: Simon and Schuster, 2008), 126.

180 "Despair shall set you free": Sontag quoted in David Rieff, *Swimming in a Sea of Death: A Son's Memoir* (New York: Simon and Schuster, 2008), 140

180 "I lived on a high horse": Sontag quoted in David Rieff, *Swimming in a Sea of Death: A Son's Memoir* (New York: Simon and Schuster, 2008), 141.

IMAGE CREDITS

PAGE 7: *Attitudes Passionnelles Extase*; photograph, 1878; Paul-Marie-Léon Regnard; J. Paul Getty Museum

PAGE 51: *Une leçon clinique à la Salpêtrière*; painting, 1887; André Brouillet; Wikimedia Commons/ Paris Descartes University

PAGE 61: *Hystéro-Épilepsie État Normal*; photograph, 1878; Paul-Marie-Léon Regnard; J. Paul Getty Museum

PAGE 63: *Attitudes Passionnelles Menace*; photograph, 1878; Paul-Marie-Léon Regnard J. Paul Getty Museum

PAGE 65: *Début d'une Attaque Cri*; photograph, 1878; Paul-Marie-Léon Regnard J. Paul Getty Museum

PAGE 67: *Loïe Fuller*; Photograph; Wikimedia Commons

PAGE 73: *The Doctor*; painting, 1891; Luke Fildes; Wikimedia Commons/ Tate National Gallery

PAGE 75: *Death in a Sickroom*; painting, 1893; painting, 1893; Edvard Much; Wikimedia Commons/ Munchmuseet

PAGE 79: *Arch of Hysteria*; Louise Bourgeois; photograph of sculpture, 1993; Wikiart

PAGE 79: *Attaque d'hystérie, homme*; photograph, c. 1859–1910; Albert Londe; Bibliothèque de Toulouse

PAGE 138: *Pinel, médecin en chef de la Salpêtrière en 1795*; painting, 1876; Tony Robert-Fleury; Wikimedia Commons

PAGE 139: *Hôpital de la Pitié-Salpétrière*; photograph, 1909; Ministère de la Culture (France)

EMILY WELLS is a writer based in Los Angeles. She holds an MFA in creative writing from UC Riverside and teaches writing at UC Irvine. She writes for publications including *Bookforum*, *Vogue*, *Interview Magazine*, *The Los Angeles Review of Books*, *The White Review*, *Flash Art*, and *Purple Fashion Magazine*. She has been a magazine editor, fashion model, crime reporter, and classically trained ballet dancer.